MCQs
and EMQs
for the
MRCS

MCQs and EMQs for the MRCS

R. AL-GHNANIEM
MRCS (Eng.)
Clinical Lecturer in Surgery,
Academic Department of Surgery,
Guy's, King's and St. Thomas' Medical School,
University of London, London, UK

I.S. BENJAMIN
BSc, MD, FRCS (Glas. and Eng.)
Professor of Surgery,
Academic Department of Surgery,
Guy's, King's and St. Thomas' Medical School,
University of London, London, UK

First published 2000

A CIP catalogue record for this book is available from the British Library.

ISBN 1 85996 118 5

BIOS Scientific Publishers Ltd
9 Newtec Place, Magdalen Road, Oxford OX4 1RE, UK
Tel. +44 (0)1865 726286. Fax. +44 (0)1865 246823
World Wide Web home page: http://www.bios.co.uk/

Important Note from the Publisher
The information contained within this book was obtained by BIOS Scientific Publishers Ltd from sources believed by us to be reliable. However, while every effort has been made to ensure its accuracy, no responsibility for loss or injury whatsoever occasioned to any person acting or refraining from action as a result of information contained herein can be accepted by the authors or publishers.

The reader should remember that medicine is a constantly evolving science and while the authors and publishers have ensured that all dosages, applications and practices are based on current indications, there may be specific practices which differ between communities. You should always follow the guidelines laid down by the manufacturers of specific products and the relevant authorities in the country in which you are practising.

Production Editor: Andrea Bosher.
Typeset by Marksbury Multimedia Ltd, Midsomer Norton, Bath, UK.
Printed by TJ International, Padstow, UK.

CONTENTS

ABBREVIATIONS

ACE	angiotensin converting enzyme
ACTH	adrenocorticotrophic hormone
AF	atrial fibrillation
AIDS	acquired immune deficiency syndrome
ALP	alkaline phosphatase
APACHE	Acute Physiology and Chronic Health Evaluation
APTT	activated partial thromboplastin time
ARDS	adult respiratory distress syndrome
AST	aspartate transaminase
ATN	acute tubular necrosis
AV	atrio-ventricular
BP	blood pressure
CO	cardiac output
COPD	chronic obstructive pulmonary disease
CPAP	continuous positive airway pressure ventilation
CSF	cerebrospinal fluid
CT	computerized tomography
CVA	cerebrovascular accident
CXR	chest X-ray
DC	direct current
DIC	disseminated intravascular coagulation
DPL	diagnostic peritoneal lavage
DSA	digital subtraction angiography
ECF	extracellular fluid
ECG	electrocardiogram
EMQ	extended matching question
ENT	ears, nose and throat
ERCP	endoscopic retrograde cholangiopancreatography
ESR	erythrocyte sedimentation rate
ESWL	extracorporeal shockwave lithotripsy
FBC	full blood count
FEV_1	forced expiratory volume in one second
FNA	fine needle aspiration
FNAC	fine needle aspiration cytology
FVC	forced vital capacity
GCS	Glasgow Coma Score
GFR	glomerular filtration rate
GTN	glyceryl trinitrate
hCG	human chorionic gonadotrophin
HIV	human immunodeficiency virus
HR	heart rate
HSV	herpes simplex virus
IA	intra-arterial

ICF	intracellular fluid
ICP	intracranial pressure
INR	international normalized ratio
IPPV	intermittent positive airway pressure ventilation
ISS	Injury Severity Score
ITS	International Trauma Score
ITU	intensive trauma unit
IV	intravenous
IVC	inferior vena cava
IVU	intravenous urogram
JVP	jugular venous pressure
MCQ	multiple choice question
MCV	mean corpuscular volume
MRI	magnetic resonance imaging
MS	multiple sclerosis
NGT	nasogastric tube
NIDDM	non-insulin dependent diabetes mellitus
NSAID	non-steroidal anti-inflammatory drug
PA	posterio-anterior
PCA	patient-controlled analgesia
PEEP	positive end expiratory pressure
PEFR	peak expiratory flow rate
PET	positron emission tomography
PIP	proximal interphalangeal
PT	prothrombin time
PTH	parathyroid hormone
RR	respiratory rate
RTS	Revised Trauma Score
SA	sino-atrial
SV	stroke volume
SVC	superior vena cava
SVR	systemic vascular resistance
TB	tuberculosis
TIA	transient ischaemic attack
TPN	total parenteral nutrition
TRH	thyrotrophin-releasing hormone
TRISS	Trauma Revised Injury Severity Score
TSH	thyroid-stimulating hormone
TURP	transurethral resection of the prostate
USS	ultrasound scan
V/Q	ventilation perfusion scan
VMA	vanilylmandelic acid
WBC	white blood cell count

PREFACE

The written part of the MRCS/AFRCS exam comprises two papers based on the 'Core' and 'System' modules set out in the syllabus. The papers are set in the Multiple Choice Questions (MCQ) and Extended Matching Questions (EMQ) format. Although Paper One is meant to cover the Core Modules and Paper Two the System Modules, there is a significant cross over of questions in the actual papers.

The papers contain 50 MCQs and 45 EMQs and are allocated 2 hours each. It is advisable that about 1 ¼ hour is spent on section 1 (MCQ) and ¾ hour on section 2 (EMQ).

In the exam you will be provided with a pencil and double-sided answer sheet (see example). Side 1 is for section 1 and side 2 for section 2. Note that the paper is not negatively marked, i.e. a correct response scores 1 and an incorrect response scores 0. It is, therefore, advisable to answer all questions.

The MCQs contain a variable number of items each of which may be true or false. You will be given an example on how to enter your answer in the answer sheet before the examination starts.

EMQs are based on a theme. You will be given a set of possible options (usually six or seven) and different scenarios. You are then asked to match the scenario with the **single most likely option**. Note that each option may be used once, more than once or not at all. Again these are not negatively marked and should all be answered.

A common problem when answering MCQs is ambiguity of certain terms. To limit this a list of definitions of common terms is given with the examination instructions as follows:

- A feature that occurs in at least 90% of cases is described as: *characteristically, classically, predominantly and reliably.*
- A feature that occurs in at least 60% of cases is described as: *typically, frequently, commonly and usually.*
- A feature that occurs in at least 30% of cases is described as: *often and tends to.*
- Terms that are deemed not to be associated with a frequency with which a feature occurs include: *recognized, associated, adequately, treatment of choice, has been shown, may be caused by and may be present.*
- *Immediate* means within 3 hours.
- *Urgent* means within 24 hours.

You will also find with the instructions a list of common abbreviations that may be used in the paper.

Reyad Al-Ghnaniem
Irving S. Benjamin

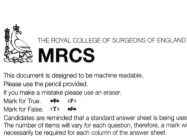

THE ROYAL COLLEGE OF SURGEONS OF ENGLAND

MRCS

This document is designed to be machine readable.
Please use the pencil provided.
If you make a mistake please use an eraser.
Mark for True.   ᴛ cF3
Mark for False.   cT3 ꜰ
Candidates are reminded that a standard answer sheet is being used.
The number of items will vary for each question, therefore, a mark will not
necessarily be required for each column of the answer sheet.

For example,
candidate 007 should
be inserted as:

0	⦿ c13 c23 c33 c43 c53 c63 c73 c83 c93
0	⦿ c13 c23 c33 c43 c53 c63 c73 c83 c93 EXAMPLE
7	c03 c13 c23 c33 c43 c53 c63 c73 c83 c93

Candidate Number

Please insert your
candidate number
as shown above.

c03 c13 c23 c33 c43 c53 c63 c73 c83 c93
c03 c13 c23 c33 c43 c53 c63 c73 c83 c93
c03 c13 c23 c33 c43 c53 c63 c73 c83 c93

Columns: A B C D E F G H (True/False bubbles for each)

Questions 1–60 with cT3 cF3 bubbles under columns A through H.

Mark Reflex® by NCSi NM-01372:   2   ED3803   Printed in U.K.   System design by Speedwell Computing Services. 01604 410041

Answer sheet reproduced with the permission of the Royal College of Surgeons

Each question will have up to ten options listed (A-J). Only one of the options will be the correct answer. Indicate your response by marking a single line through the appropriate box.

For example:

Question 61 correct answer is option C
Question 62 correct answer is option F
Question 63 correct answer is option A

	A	B	C	D	E	F	G	H	I	J
61	cA3	cB3	━●━	cD3	cE3	cF3	cG3	cH3	c I 3	cJ3
62	cA3	cB3	cC3	cD3	cE3	━F━	cG3	cH3	c I 3	cJ3
63	━A━	cB3	cC3	cD3	cE3	cF3	cG3	cH3	c I 3	cJ3

	A	B	C	D	E	F	G	H	I	J			A	B	C	D	E	F	G	H	I	J
61	cA3	cB3	cC3	cD3	cE3	cF3	cG3	cH3	c I 3	cJ3		111	cA3	cB3	cC3	cD3	cE3	cF3	cG3	cH3	c I 3	cJ3
62	cA3	cB3	cC3	cD3	cE3	cF3	cG3	cH3	c I 3	cJ3		112	cA3	cB3	cC3	cD3	cE3	cF3	cG3	cH3	c I 3	cJ3
63	cA3	cB3	cC3	cD3	cE3	cF3	cG3	cH3	c I 3	cJ3		113	cA3	cB3	cC3	cD3	cE3	cF3	cG3	cH3	c I 3	cJ3
64	cA3	cB3	cC3	cD3	cE3	cF3	cG3	cH3	c I 3	cJ3		114	cA3	cB3	cC3	cD3	cE3	cF3	cG3	cH3	c I 3	cJ3
65	cA3	cB3	cC3	cD3	cE3	cF3	cG3	cH3	c I 3	cJ3		115	cA3	cB3	cC3	cD3	cE3	cF3	cG3	cH3	c I 3	cJ3
66	cA3	cB3	cC3	cD3	cE3	cF3	cG3	cH3	c I 3	cJ3		116	cA3	cB3	cC3	cD3	cE3	cF3	cG3	cH3	c I 3	cJ3
67	cA3	cB3	cC3	cD3	cE3	cF3	cG3	cH3	c I 3	cJ3		117	cA3	cB3	cC3	cD3	cE3	cF3	cG3	cH3	c I 3	cJ3
68	cA3	cB3	cC3	cD3	cE3	cF3	cG3	cH3	c I 3	cJ3		118	cA3	cB3	cC3	cD3	cE3	cF3	cG3	cH3	c I 3	cJ3
69	cA3	cB3	cC3	cD3	cE3	cF2	cG3	cH3	c I 3	cJ3		119	cA3	cB3	cC3	cD3	cE3	cF3	cG3	cH3	c I 3	cJ3
70	cA3	cB3	cC3	cD3	cE3	cF3	cG3	cH3	c I 3	cJ3		120	cA3	cB3	cC3	cD3	cE3	cF3	cG3	cH3	c I 3	cJ3
71	cA3	cB3	cC3	cD3	cE3	cF2	cG3	cH3	c I 3	cJ3		121	cA3	cB3	cC3	cD3	cE3	cF3	cG3	cH3	c I 3	cJ3
72	cA3	cB3	cC3	cD3	cE3	cF2	cG3	cH3	c I 3	cJ3		122	cA3	cB3	cC3	cD3	cE3	cF3	cG3	cH3	c I 3	cJ3
73	cA3	cB3	cC3	cD3	cE3	cF3	cG3	cH3	c I 3	cJ3		123	cA3	cB3	cC3	cD3	cE3	cF3	cG3	cH3	c I 3	cJ3
74	cA3	cB3	cC3	cD3	cE3	cF3	cG3	cH3	c I 3	cJ3		124	cA3	cB3	cC3	cD3	cE3	cF3	cG3	cH3	c I 3	cJ3
75	cA3	cB3	cC2	cD3	cE3	cF3	cG3	cH3	c I 3	cJ3		125	cA3	cB3	cC3	cD3	cE3	cF3	cG3	cH3	c I 3	cJ3
76	cA3	cB3	cC2	cD3	cE3	cF3	cG3	cH3	c I 3	cJ3		126	cA3	cB3	cC3	cD3	cE3	cF3	cG3	cH3	c I 3	cJ3
77	cA3	cB3	cC2	cD3	cE3	cF3	cG3	cH3	c I 3	cJ3		127	cA3	cB3	cC3	cD3	cE3	cF3	cG3	cH3	c I 3	cJ3
78	cA3	cB3	cC2	cD3	cE3	cF2	cG3	cH3	c I 3	cJ3		128	cA3	cB3	cC2	cD3	cE3	cF3	cG3	cH3	c I 3	cJ3
79	cA3	cB3	cC2	cD3	cE3	cF3	cG3	cH3	c I 3	cJ3		129	cA3	cB3	cC2	cD3	cE3	cF3	cG3	cH3	c I 3	cJ3
80	cA3	cB3	cC2	cD3	cE3	cF3	cG3	cH3	c I 3	cJ3		130	cA3	cB3	cC3	cD3	cE3	cF3	cG3	cH3	c I 3	cJ3
81	cA3	cB3	cC2	cD3	cE3	cF3	cG3	cH3	c I 3	cJ3		131	cA3	cB3	cC2	cD3	cE3	cF3	cG3	cH3	c I 3	cJ3
82	cA3	cB3	cC2	cD3	cE3	cF3	cG3	cH3	c I 3	cJ3		132	cA3	cB3	cC3	cD3	cE3	cF3	cG3	cH3	c I 3	cJ3
83	cA3	cB3	cC2	cD3	cE3	cF3	cG3	cH3	c I 3	cJ3		133	cA3	cB3	cC3	cD3	cE3	cF3	cG3	cH3	c I 3	cJ3
84	cA3	cB3	cC2	cD3	cE3	cF3	cG3	cH3	c I 3	cJ3		134	cA3	cB3	cC2	cD3	cE3	cF3	cG3	cH3	c I 3	cJ3
85	cA3	cB3	cC2	cD3	cE3	cF3	cG3	cH3	c I 3	cJ3		135	cA3	cB3	cC3	cD3	cE3	cF3	cG3	cH3	c I 3	cJ3
86	cA3	cB3	cC2	cD3	cE3	cF3	cG3	cH3	c I 3	cJ3		136	cA3	cB3	cC3	cD3	cE3	cF3	cG3	cH3	c I 3	cJ3
87	cA3	cB3	cC2	cD3	cE3	cF3	cG3	cH3	c I 3	cJ3		137	cA3	cB3	cC3	cD3	cE3	cF3	cG3	cH3	c I 3	cJ3
88	cA3	cB3	cC2	cD3	cE3	cF3	cG3	cH3	c I 3	cJ3		138	cA3	cB3	cC3	cD3	cE3	cF3	cG3	cH3	c I 3	cJ3
89	cA3	cB3	cC2	cD3	cE3	cF3	cG3	cH3	c I 3	cJ3		139	cA3	cB3	cC3	cD3	cE3	cF3	cG3	cH3	c I 3	cJ3
90	cA3	cB3	cC2	cD3	cE3	cF3	cG3	cH3	c I 3	cJ3		140	cA3	cB3	cC3	cD3	cE3	cF3	cG3	cH3	c I 3	cJ3
91	cA3	cB3	cC2	cD3	cE3	cF3	cG3	cH3	c I 3	cJ3		141	cA3	cB3	cC3	cD3	cE3	cF3	cG3	cH3	c I 3	cJ3
92	cA3	cB3	cC2	cD3	cE3	cF3	cG3	cH3	c I 3	cJ3		142	cA3	cB3	cC2	cD3	cE3	cF3	cG3	cH3	c I 3	cJ3
93	cA3	cB3	cC2	cD3	cE3	cF3	cG3	cH3	c I 3	cJ3		143	cA3	cB3	cC3	cD3	cE3	cF3	cG3	cH3	c I 3	cJ3
94	cA3	cB3	cC3	cD3	cE3	cF3	cG3	cH3	c I 3	cJ3		144	cA3	cB3	cC3	cD3	cE3	cF3	cG3	cH3	c I 3	cJ3
95	cA3	cB3	cC3	cD3	cE3	cF3	cG3	cH3	c I 3	cJ3		145	cA3	cB3	cC2	cD3	cE3	cF3	cG3	cH3	c I 3	cJ3
96	cA3	cB3	cC3	cD3	cE3	cF3	cG3	cH3	c I 3	cJ3		146	cA3	cB3	cC3	cD3	cE3	cF3	cG3	cH3	c I 3	cJ3
97	cA3	cB3	cC3	cD3	cE3	cF3	cG3	cH3	c I 3	cJ3		147	cA3	cB3	cC3	cD3	cE3	cF3	cG3	cH3	c I 3	cJ3
98	cA3	cB3	cC3	cD2	cE3	cF3	cG3	cH3	c I 3	cJ3		148	cA3	cB3	cC3	cD3	cE3	cF3	cG3	cH3	c I 3	cJ3
99	cA3	cB3	cC3	cD3	cE3	cF3	cG3	cH3	c I 3	cJ3		149	cA3	cB3	cC3	cD3	cE3	cF3	cG3	cH3	c I 3	cJ3
100	cA3	cB3	cC3	cD3	cE3	cF3	cG3	cH3	c I 3	cJ3		150	cA3	cB3	cC3	cD3	cE3	cF3	cG3	cH3	c I 3	cJ3
101	cA3	cB3	cC3	cD3	cE3	cF3	cG3	cH3	c I 3	cJ3		151	cA3	cB3	cC2	cD3	cE3	cF3	cG3	cH3	c I 3	cJ3
102	cA3	cB3	cC3	cD3	cE3	cF2	cG3	cH3	c I 3	cJ3		152	cA3	cB3	cC3	cD3	cE3	cF3	cG3	cH3	c I 3	cJ3
103	cA3	cB3	cC3	cD3	cE3	cF3	cG3	cH3	c I 3	cJ3		153	cA3	cB3	cC3	cD3	cE3	cF3	cG3	cH3	c I 3	cJ3
104	cA3	cB3	cC3	cD3	cE3	cF3	cG3	cH3	c I 3	cJ3		154	cA3	cB3	cC2	cD3	cE3	cF3	cG3	cH3	c I 3	cJ3
105	cA3	cB3	cC2	cD3	cE3	cF3	cG3	cH3	c I 3	cJ3		155	cA3	cB3	cC3	cD3	cE3	cF3	cG3	cH3	c I 3	cJ3
106	cA3	cB3	cC2	cD3	cE3	cF3	cG3	cH3	c I 3	cJ3		156	cA3	cB3	cC3	cD3	cE3	cF3	cG3	cH3	c I 3	cJ3
107	cA3	cB3	cC2	cD3	cE3	cF3	cG3	cH3	c I 3	cJ3		157	cA3	cB3	cC3	cD3	cE3	cF3	cG3	cH3	c I 3	cJ3
108	cA3	cB3	cC3	cD3	cE3	cF3	cG2	cH3	c I 3	cJ3		158	cA3	cB3	cC3	cD3	cE3	cF3	cG3	cH3	c I 3	cJ3
109	cA3	cB3	cC3	cD3	cE3	cF3	cG3	cH3	c I 3	cJ3		159	cA3	cB3	cC3	cD3	cE3	cF3	cG3	cH3	c I 3	cJ3
110	cA3	cB3	cC3	cD3	cE3	cF3	cG3	cH3	c I 3	cJ3		160	cA3	cB3	cC3	cD3	cE3	cF3	cG3	cH3	c I 3	cJ3

FOREWORD

Surgical examinations in the UK have undergone a remarkable and timely 'quiet revolution' in recent years. The days of the 'Primary' and 'Final' Fellowship examinations in general surgery, which were sat after a training period of variable length, and varied experience, have gone and have been replaced by a 2 year structured educational programme at the senior house officer level, which culminates in the MRCS or AFRCS examination. This period of basic training precedes entry to specialty training and final assessment in any one of 14 specialty examinations offered by the Intercollegiate Examinations Board.

The examination departments of the four Surgical Colleges have modified the tests of clinical competence in their examinations which have now become more uniform in their format. The topics of vivas have also been defined and tested to improve the objectivity of assessments in knowledge and communication skills. It is intended that these changes will provide an even standard in the examination process for all trainees.

The revolution in examination techniques has particularly affected the written parts of examinations, in which Multiple Choice Questions are now so prominent. MCQs were pioneered in the United States more than 50 years ago with the avowed purpose of introducing an objective method of testing knowledge, thus removing the variation in subjective judgement which is inherent in the marking of the traditional essay-type questions, (although the latter can still be defended as valuable tests in the skills of comprehension, organization, logic, and creativity).

It is advisable for surgical trainees to have some practical experience of the type of questions which they will encounter in the new surgical examinations and I can recommend this book as a useful guide for both the MRCS and AFRCS papers. Furthermore, the perusal of MCQ's can provide a personal measure of educational attainment and a relatively painless method of absorbing facts.

The construction of MCQs, and their various modifications, is an arduous task and I congratulate the authors of this volume on the range of topics and their skill in question construction. I believe that the book could be a sound investment for the surgical tyro.

Edward R Howard MS FRCS(Eng) FRCS(Edin)
Professor Emeritus in Hepatobiliary Surgery
King's College Hospital
London SE5 9RS

Acknowledgements

We would like to thank Maria Pufulete for editing the original manuscript, Mr Joseph Perez for reviewing the orthopaedics section, Mr Peter Carroll for his valuable suggestions, Miss Caroline O'Leary for her secretarial work and Sanjay Gupta. We would also like to thank the staff at BIOS for being efficient and patient.

PRACTICE PAPER ONE: CORE MODULES

MCQs

1. **Rectal prolapse**

    A   Is associated with reduced anal tone
    B   May be treated with a Delorme's procedure
    C   In adults is more common in females
    D   In children is treated with rectopexy

2. **Malignant melanoma**

    A   Is staged histologically using Clarke's level
    B   Carries best prognosis when less than 5 mm deep
    C   Is most commonly 'superficial spreading' in type
    D   Carries a poor prognosis when it affects the squamous mucosa
    E   Metastasizes to the viscera

3. **Continuous positive airway pressure ventilation (CPAP)**

    A   Increases the peak expiratory flow rate
    B   Increases the functional residual capacity
    C   Improves V/Q mismatch
    D   Improves oxygenation in atelectasis
    E   Reduces the work of respiration

4. **The following increase cardiac contractility**

    A   Increased preload
    B   Vagus activity
    C   Phrenic nerve activity
    D   Adrenaline
    E   Glucagon
    F   Mild to moderate hypoxia

5. **Crush syndrome**

A   Is associated with hyperkalaemia
B   Myoglobinaemia may produce acute tubular necrosis
C   There is hypocalcaemia
D   Carries a very high mortality in the presence of established acute renal failure
E   May occur secondary to drug overdose

6. **In managing the traumatized patient**

A   A large intravenous cannula is needed
B   The airway is secured after assessing the patient's conscious level
C   Cervical spine injury may be excluded if neurological examination is normal
D   Profuse bleeding from a limb should be arrested by applying a tourniquet
E   The patient should not be exposed to prevent hypothermia

7. **Fluid requirement**

A   Is about 2.5 l per day in an average subject
B   Varies according to the ambient temperature
C   Is met by replacing gastrointestinal losses with 5% dextrose solution
D   Should be doubled in the burned patient
E   Is higher, per kilogram of weight, in the child compared with adults

8. **Regarding local anaesthetics**

A   Bupivicaine is the least cardiotoxic
B   Prilocaine is used in Bier's block
C   The maximum allowed dose of plain lignocaine is 10 mg/kg
D   Produce anaesthesia by blocking Na–K channels
E   An overdose presents with sudden loss of consciousness and coma

9. **The following are DNA viruses**

A   Hepatitis A
B   Hepatitis B
C   Hepatitis C
D   HIV
E   Herpes simplex

10. **Liver trauma**

A   Is uncommon compared to other abdominal organs
B   May be complicated by liver embolism
C   Is treated with liver resection to control bleeding
D   Can be treated conservatively by embolizing the bleeding vessel
E   Haemobilia may be a late consequence

11. **Regarding antibiotic prophylaxis in surgery**

A   It should be used as a 3-day course
B   The maximum plasma concentration should be achieved within the hour before surgery
C   Antibiotics with the widest possible spectrum should be used
D   It is not needed in upper digestive tract surgery
E   It does not reduce the risk of wound infection in gangrenous appendicitis

12. **The following are absorbable sutures**

A   Cat gut
B   Polyamide
C   Polydioxanone
D   Polyglactin
E   Silk
F   Polytetrafluoroethylene

13. *Clostridium tetani*

A   Is Gram-negative
B   Produces a toxin called tetanospasmin
C   Causes gangrene only in the presence of *Proteus*
D   Infection is prevented by a vaccination that needs to be repeated every 2 years
E   Neuromuscular blockade and ventilation is part of the management in fulminant infection

14. **The following are contraindications to spinal anaesthesia**

A   .Coagulopathy
B   Alzheimer's disease
C   Pilonidal abscess
D   Multiple sclerosis
E   Operations for acute haemorrhage

15. **The nerves most commonly injured during patient handling in theatre include**

A Femoral
B Ulnar
C Common peroneal
D Saphenous
E The brachial plexus

16. **Abdominal wound dehiscence**

A Is usually heralded by bleeding from the wound
B Is a recognized risk in the jaundiced patient
C Occurs 5–10 days postoperatively
D Occurs more commonly in those having surgery for malignant conditions
E Is best avoided by following Jenkins' rule, i.e. the length of the suture should be at least twice that of the wound

17. **The following are used to assess fluid status**

A Skin turgor
B Pulse oximetry
C Central venous pressure
D White cell count
E Change in haematocrit

18. **The following blood products are derived from more than one donor**

A Albumin
B Red blood cells
C Whole blood
D Fresh frozen plasma
E Platelets
F Coagulation factor concentrate

19. **Obesity in surgical patients is associated with the following**

A Wound dehiscence
B Venous thromboembolism
C Respiratory tract infections
D Bleeding disorders
E Altered pharmacokinetics of anaesthetic drugs

20. **The following clotting factors are vitamin K dependent**

A   II
B   III
C   V
D   VII
E   VIII
F   IX
G   X

21. **Venous anatomy**

A   The left brachiocephalic vein forms behind the left sternoclavicular joint
B   the superior vena cava commences behind the 1st right costosternal joint
C   The azygos vein drains into the right brachiocephalic vein
D   The inferior vena cava has an intrathoracic course about 7 cm long
E   The left superior intercostal vein drains into the left brachiocephalic vein

22. **Smokers have increased risk of postoperative pneumonia due to**

A   Viscid secretions
B   Reduced immunity
C   Obesity
D   Loss of cilia in the respiratory tract
E   Inability to cough

23. **Surgical trauma has the following metabolic effects**

A   Hyponatraemia
B   Hypoglycaemia
C   Increased cortisol levels
D   Increased total body water
E   Increased metabolic rate

24. **Type IV or delayed hypersensitivity**

A   Is cell mediated
B   Is implicated in graft rejection
C   Is the mechanism by which rheumatoid arthritis develops
D   The effect occurs 1 hour after onset of reaction
E   Is thought to occur in Hashimoto's thyroiditis

25. **The following protective clothing is mandatory for a trauma team member**

A   Goggles
B   Face masks
C   Sterile surgical gowns
D   Gloves
E   Aprons

26. **Regarding disseminated intravascular coagulation**

A   It may be caused by massive trauma
B   There is elevated plasma fibrinogen
C   Thrombocytopenia is an early feature
D   It is treated with an infusion of heparin
E   It may present with widespread thrombosis

27. **The following are features of cardiac tamponade**

A   Elevated JVP
B   Kussmaul's sign
D   Split-second heart sound
E   Hypotension
F   Increased cardiac output

28. **Regarding the traumatized child**

A   The systolic blood pressure can be estimated as twice the child's age plus 80 mmHg
B   Initial resuscitation is with warmed crystalloid in a dose of 20 ml/kg
C   Visceral damage is highly unlikely in the absence of external injuries
D   Diagnostic peritoneal lavage should be employed in the first instance where visceral injury is suspected

29. **A fracture through the angle of the mandible displaces**

A   The tongue backwards
B   The ramus backwards
C   The ramus medially
D   The ramus upwards
E   The ramus forwards
F   The zygomatic arch downwards

30. Anatomy of the heart

A   The coronary sinuses arise distal to the right and left aortic valvules
B   The posterior descending artery is a branch of the left coronary artery
C   Coronary venous blood mainly drains directly into the heart chambers
D   The cardiac veins drain into the superior vena cava
E   The left ventricle receives some of its blood supply from the right coronary artery
F   The right coronary artery branches usually supply the SA and AV nodes

31. Recognized indications for emergency laparotomy in a trauma patient

A   Gunshot wound
B   Free air in the peritoneum on X-ray
C   Unexplained shock in the traumatized patient
D   After positive diagnostic peritoneal lavage
E   Left lower ribs fracture and overlying bruising

32. Valsalva manoeuvre

A   Generates high intrathoracic pressure
B   Increases the cardiac output
C   Causes peripheral vasoconstriction
D   Produces reflex bradycardia after termination of the manoeuvre
E   May terminate a supraventricular tachycardia

33. Phrenic nerves

A   Arise from the dorsal rami of C3–C5
B   Lie anterior to the vagus throughout their thoracic course
C   Supply sensory fibres to the pericardium
D   The right nerve pierces the diaphragm with the IVC
E   Pass posterior to the lung hila

34. In the cardiac cycle

A   The 'a' wave of the jugular vein corresponds with the PR interval on the ECG
B   Aortic valve closure corresponds with the 2nd heart sound
C   The QRS complex corresponds with the 2nd heart sound
D   Blood flow across the aortic valve commences after the S wave on ECG
E   A very large jugular 'v' wave is associated with mitral regurgitation

35. **Methods of delivering 100% inspired oxygen to patients**

A 201 O_2 through face mask
B CPAP
C Tracheostomy
D Endotracheal intubation
E Needle cricothyroidotomy

36. **Hepatic encephalopathy**

A Is due to portosystemic shunting
B Is precipitated by fresh rectal bleeding
C May be improved by purgatives
D May be precipitated by hyponatraemia
E Is precipitated by spontaneous bacterial peritonitis

37. **Typical features of a malignant neoplasm**

A De-differentiation
B Small nucleus and large cytoplasm
C Increased number of abnormal mitoses
D Pleomorphism
E Hypochromatic nucleus

38. **The following factors enhance angiogenesis of metastases**

A Epidermal growth factor
B Tumour necrosis factor α
C Angiostatin
D Transforming growth factor α
E Transforming growth factor β

39. **Fat necrosis of the breast**

A Produces a hard lump mimicking carcinoma
B Is easily diagnosed in the presence of clear history of trauma
C May produce skin tethering
D Typically presents with inflammation
E Nipple retraction does not occur

40. **Neurofibromatosis**

A   Is associated with acoustic neuroma
B   Has an autosomal dominant inheritance
C   Presents in childhood
D   May be associated with café-au-lait spots
E   The neurofibromas have no malignant potential

41. **Brain tumours**

A   Are responsible for 10% of all deaths
B   Secondary metastases are more common in the elderly
C   Supratentorial tumours are more common in childhood
D   May present with diplopia
E   Of the corpus callosum present with dementia and incontinence

42. **Bilirubin**

A   Is also known as deoxycholic acid
B   Is a metabolite of cholesterol
C   Is converted to urobilinogen in the hepatocyte
D   Jaundice is detected when the serum concentration is above about $30\,\mu mol/l$
E   Obstructive jaundice is unlikely in the presence of high levels of urobilinogen in the urine

43. **The following are recognized urachal abnormalities**

A   Urachal cyst
B   Urachal diverticulum
C   External urachal sinus
D   Patent urachus
E   Vesicoenteric fistula

44. **Carcinoma of the gall bladder**

A   Is common in South American Indians
B   Does not present with jaundice
C   The treatment may involve right hepatic lobectomy
D   Surgical treatment does not improve prognosis
E   Is more common in males

45. **Indications for preoperative chest X-ray (CXR) include**

A   Known history of COPD
B   Age over 55 years
C   Ivor–Lewis oesophagectomy
D   A 32-year-old patient undergoing orchidectomy for testicular cancer
E   Coronary artery bypass graft

46. **The following are common indications for inserting a central venous catheter**

A   Replacement of large volumes of fluid in a short period
B   Cardiac pacemaker
C   Pneumothorax
D   Monitoring right heart function
E   Infusion of certain drugs

47. **Long-term dialysis is associated with**

A   Sarcoidosis
B β2 amyloidosis
C   Renal osteodystrophy
D   Anaemia
E   Acquired multicystic kidney disease

48. **Pneumatic anti-shock garments**

A   Are used to treat a haemothorax
B   Reduce the functioning volume of the vascular compartment
C   Can be used to splint a femoral fracture
D   Have a haemodynamic effect equivalent to transfusing > 1 l of blood
E   May be safely used in cases with diaphragmatic rupture

49. **Lung compliance**

A   Is inversely related to change in pressure
B   Is high when increases in lung volume are easy to achieve
C   Is reduced in ARDS
D   Is reduced by increased intra-abdominal pressure

50. **Regarding intracranial pressure (ICP)**

A   It is inversely related to cerebral perfusion pressure
B   Hypercapnia increases ICP
C   It depends on the amount of CSF in the cranium
D   It produces hypotension and tachycardia if abnormally elevated
E   High ICP produces respiratory failure
F   Increased ICP may result in transtentorial herniation

EMQs

Theme: Skin lesions

Options:
a   Cavernous angioma
b   Squamous cell carcinoma
c   Keratoacanthoma
d   Melanoma
e   Basal cell carcinoma
f   Solar keratosis
g   Dermatofibroma

For each of the case scenarios below, choose the single most likely option from the list above. Each option may be used once, more than once or not at all.

61. A 74-year-old retired builder presents with a long-standing and slowly enlarging skin lesion on his right cheek. On examination this appears pearly with telangiectasia.
62. The parents of a 3-week-old baby are concerned as she has developed a fleshy red lesion on her face.
63. A 37-year-old executive presents with an itchy brown lesion on her left leg which sometimes bleeds.
64. The GP of a 68-year-old woman refers her to the surgical outpatients with a month's history of a skin lesion which has developed on her face. Three months have passed and by the time she attends her appointment the lesion has disappeared.

Theme: Anaemia

Options:
a   Iron deficiency anaemia
b   Spherocytosis
c B_{12} deficiency anaemia
d   β thalassaemia

e   Sickle cell disease
f   Glucose-6-phosphate dehydrogenase deficiency
g   Sideroblastic anaemia
h   Pernicious anaemia

For each of the case scenarios below, choose the single most likely option from the list above. Each option may be used once, more than once or not at all.

65. An 11-year-old Caucasian girl of Scottish origin presents with mild anaemia and jaundice. The MCV is normal but the red cell osmotic fragility is increased.
66. A patient presents with severe back pain. He is 25 and of African origin. Investigations reveal normocytic, normochromic anaemia, high reticulocyte count and jaundice. The ESR is low.
67. A man presents with shortness of breath and worsening angina. On examination he has an upper midline incision for an ulcer operation several years ago. His FBC shows macrocytic anaemia and his Schilling test is negative.

Theme: Prophylactic antibiotics

Options:
a   Cefuroxime
b   Gentamicin
c   Amoxycillin
d   Ciprofloxacin and metronidazole
e   Metronidazole
f   Ciprofloxacin and amoxycillin
g   a&c
h   a&e

For each of the case scenarios below, choose the single most likely option from the list above. Each option may be used once, more than once or not at all.

68. Total knee replacement.
69. Right hemicolectomy.
70. A patient undergoing ERCP for stones in common bile duct.

Theme: Fluid replacement in 24 hours

Options:
a   3l of dextrose/saline
b   3l of 0.9% saline
c   1.5l of 5% dextrose
d   3l of dextrose/saline and 1l of 0.9% saline
e   1.5l of 0.9% saline
f   3l of gelatin solution

g 2 l of 5% dextrose and 3 l of 0.9% saline
h 2 l of 0.9% saline

For each of the case scenarios below, choose the single most likely option from the list above. Each option may be used once, more than once or not at all.

71. A patient is admitted with gastric outlet obstruction. The nasogastric aspirate is 2 l per 24 hours.
72. A 55-year-old patient who is known to be an alcoholic presents with progressive ascites and oedema. His weight has increased by 7 kg and his serum sodium is 120 mmol/l.
73. A 35-year-old male with ulcerative colitis underwent subtotal colectomy and ileostomy formation. Postoperatively the patient develops an enterocutaneous fistula which produces 2 l of effluent per day. He receives 2.5 l of TPN.

Theme: Chest pain

Options:
a Myocardial infarction
b Pulmonary embolus
c Pneumonia
d Tietz's syndrome
e Pneumothorax
f Oesophegeal spasm
g Dissecting aneurysm

For each of the case scenarios below, choose the single most likely option from the list above. Each option may be used once, more than once or not at all.

74. A 57-year-old man attends A&E describing a crushing retrosternal chest pain which radiates to the jaw. He has had this pain intermittently for 3 years. A coronary angiogram 3 months ago was normal.
75. A 37-year-old woman presents 2 weeks postpartum with pleuritic chest pain, shortness of breath and haemoptysis.
76. A 17-year-old female with a history of asthma and epilepsy presents with anterior chest pain and shortness of breath. The anterior chest wall is tender on percussion.

Theme: Blood transfusion

Options:
a A RhD positive
b A RhD negative
c B RhD positive
d O RhD positive
e AB RhD positive

f   AB RhD negative

g   O RhD negative

For each of the case scenarios below, choose the single most likely option from the list above. Each option may be used once, more than once or not at all.

77. A woman, in her early thirties, with blood group B RhD negative needs transfusion.
78. A patient with blood group AB RhD positive requires fresh frozen plasma.
79. A 55-year-old man with blood group B RhD negative needs transfusion. The blood bank has a severe shortage of O RhD negative.

Theme: Glasgow Coma Scale (GCS)

Options:

a   5

b   6

c   7

d   8

e   9

f   10

g   11

For each of the case scenarios below, choose the single most likely option from the list above. Each option may be used once, more than once or not at all.

80. Eyes open to speech, flexes to pain and confused speech.
81. Eyes open to pain, localizes to pain and inappropriate words.
82. Eyes do not open, extends to pain and produces incomprehensible sounds.

Theme: Haemorrhagic shock

Options:

a   Class I

b   Class I a

c   Class II

d   Class II b

e   Class III

f   Class IV

g   Class V

For each of the case scenarios below, choose the single most likely option from the list above. Each option may be used once, more than once or not at all.

83. A 35-year-old man with a pulse rate of 110 bpm and a BP of 120/94 mmHg.
84. A 42-year-old woman with an estimated blood loss of 2 l.
85. A 19-year-old man with a very weak pulse of 140 bpm and BP of 55/30 mmHg. He is unconscious, ashen and cold.

Theme: The inflamed or swollen breast

Options:
a   Peau d'orange
b   Mastitis
c   Breast abscess
d   Seroma
e   Inflammatory carcinoma
f   Tubular carcinoma
g   Galactocoele

For each of the case scenarios below, choose the single most likely option from the list above. Each option may be used once, more than once or not at all.

86. A woman presents 3 weeks postpartum with a painful swelling of her right breast. On examination the breast is inflamed but there was no evidence of a mass.

87. A woman presents with painless enlargement of the right breast 6 weeks after she gave birth to a child with a cleft palate. On examination the breast is enlarged, non-tender and there are no signs of inflammation.

88. An elderly woman presents with a hard breast lump. The overlying skin is red and hot.

Theme: Management of abdominal trauma

Options:
a   Emergency laparotomy
b   Diagnostic peritoneal lavage
c   Ultrasound scan
d   Wound exploration under local anaesthetic
e   CT scan
f   Angiogram
g   Observation

For each of the case scenarios below, choose the single most likely option from the list above. Each option may be used once, more than once or not at all.

89. A young man is brought into hospital with an abdominal stab wound. The wound appears superficial, and his abdomen is soft. The pulse is 110 bpm and BP 120/80 mmHg.

90. A 32-year-old female involved in a motorcycle accident is unconscious with severe head injury. A left pneumothorax was treated with a chest drain and her pulse is 115 bpm and BP is 110/75 mmHg after 2 l of crystalloids. The abdomen is soft but otherwise difficult to assess.

91. A young man sustains a low energy transfer gunshot wound from a close range to his hypogastric area. His pulse is 130 bpm and BP 100/65 mmHg.

Theme: Lumps and bumps

Options:
a   Sebaceous cyst
b   Dermoid cyst
c   Histiocytoma
d   Ivory osteoma
e   Lipoma
f   Ganglion
g   Neurofibroma

For each of the case scenarios below, choose the single most likely option from the list above. Each option may be used once, more than once or not at all.

92.   A 1.5 cm swelling above the outer canthus. On examination it feels soft and deep to the skin with no deep attachment.
93.   A 37-year-old man presents with a 2 cm lump on the forehead which has been present for many years. On examination it feels hard and deep to the skin.
94.   A 1 cm cutaneous lump on the front of the leg which developed following an insect bite about a year previously.

Theme: Causes of reduced urine output

Options:
a   Interstitial nephritis
b   Acute glomerulonephritis
c   Urinary outflow obstruction
d   Shock-induced ATN
e   Toxic ATN
f   Haemolytic uraemic syndrome
g   Hypovolaemia

For each of the case scenarios below, choose the single most likely option from the list above. Each option may be used once, more than once or not at all.

95.   Oliguria in a patient 1 day postgastrectomy. Investigations reveal Ur 14 mmol/l, Cr 110 mmol/l, K 5 mmol/l and urinary sodium 7 mmol/l.
96.   Oliguria in a patient following coronary bypass grafting. Ur 18 mmol/l, Cr 180 mmol/l, K 5.5 mmol/l and urinary sodium 70 mmol/l.

Theme: Management of intestinal polyps

Options:
a   Abdominoperineal resection
b   Anterior resection
c   Endoscopic excision

d   No treatment is required
e   Pan-proctocolectomy
f   Subtotal colectomy
g   Regular endoscopic surveillance
h   Restorative proctocolectomy

For each of the case scenarios below, choose the single most likely option from the list above. Each option may be used once, more than once or not at all.

97. A patient with long-standing ulcerative colitis affecting the whole colon is found to have malignancy on a biopsy taken 5 cm from the anal verge and severe dysplasia on other biopsies of the rest of the colon.
98. An elderly patient presents with rectal bleeding. She is known to have haemorrhoids but rigid sigmoidoscopy revealed a small polyp 14 cm from the anal margin. A barium enema was normal and the histology shows a metaplastic polyp.
99. A 35-year-old patient with familial adenomatous polyposis presents with severely dysplastic changes in the sigmoid colon.

Theme: Staging of cancer

Options:
a   Dukes' A
b   Dukes' B
c   Dukes' C
d   Clarke's level I
e   Clarke's level II
f   Clarke's level IV
g   Clarke's level V

For each of the case scenarios below, choose the single most likely option from the list above. Each option may be used once, more than once or not at all.

100. A sigmoid colon tumour with involved circumferential margins but no lymph node deposits.
101. A melanoma invading the papillary dermis.
102. A melanoma invading the subcutaneous tissue.

Theme: Management of breast conditions

Options:
a   Wide local excision
b   Radical mastectomy
c   Chemotherapy
d   Subcutaneous mastectomy
e   Tamoxifen
f   Radiotherapy
g   Wide local excision and axillary clearance

For each of the case scenarios below, choose the single most likely option from the list above. Each option may be used once, more than once or not at all.

103. A woman in her early fifties presents with a 2 cm tumour and no axillary lymphadenopathy.

104. A 92-year-old woman presents with a slowly enlarging lump in the right breast. This proves to be a carcinoma on biopsy.

105. A 17-year-old male presents with unilateral tender enlargement of the breast for 6 months. There has been no change in size, but the swelling is causing him embarrassment and pain.

ANSWERS TO PRACTICE PAPER ONE

The letters of the correct answers are given

MCQs

1. Rectal prolapse

A, B, C

This condition is best treated with toilet training and laxatives in children. Some may require injection sclerotherapy.

2. Malignant melanoma

A, C, D, E

A thickness of less than 0.75 mm carries the best prognosis.

3. Continuous positive airway pressure ventilation (CPAP)

B, C, D, E

4. The following increase cardiac contractility

A, D, E, F

The vagus has a negative inotropic effect on the heart. The phrenic has no effect on cardiac contractility. Severe hypoxia has a negative inotropic effect.

5. Crush syndrome

A, B, D, E

Crush syndrome occurs with massive soft tissue injury and necrosis. This may be traumatic or secondary to prolonged coma as occurs in drug overdose. The necrotic tissue releases potassium, myoglobin and other products which cause the systemic effects in this syndrome.

6. In managing the traumatized patient

All false

The patient's airway is assessed first with control of the cervical spine. Cervical spine injury cannot be excluded on clinical grounds alone and multiple X-ray views are needed before immobilization is discontinued. At least two large-bore intravenous canulae are needed for resuscitation, and bleeding must be stopped with manual pressure if possible. The application of a tourniquet is not recommended. Exposure is necessary for performing a thorough examination.

7. Fluid requirement

A, B, E

Gastrointestinal secretions have a similar electrolyte content to plasma and are replaced with 0.9% saline with added potassium.

There are different formulae to calculate the fluid requirement in patients with burns, which is closely related to the surface area burned.

8. Regarding local anaesthetics
B, D
Prilocaine is the least cardiotoxic if inadvertently injected into a vein, making it a natural choice for Bier's block. Knowledge of the maximum allowed dose of the different agents helps to avoid overdose: this is 3 mg/kg for lignocaine and 7 mg/kg when mixed with adrenaline. The neurotoxic effect of an overdose manifests in epileptic fits followed ultimately by coma.

9. The following are DNA viruses
B, E
The others are RNA viruses.

10. Liver trauma
B, D, E
The liver is one of the most commonly injured organs. The treatment should be as conservative as possible and is a combination of interventional radiology, packing, tissue sealants and ligation of bleeding vessels. Liver resection should be avoided if possible as it carries a high mortality.

11. Regarding antibiotic prophylaxis in surgery
All false
Prophylactic antibiotics should be given as a single dose in most cases. The time of administration is chosen in order to achieve maximum plasma concentration at the time of surgery. The narrowest spectrum antibiotic which can cover the infecting organisms should be used.

12. The following are absorbable sutures
A, C, D

13. *Clostridium tetani*
B, E
C. tetani is an anaerobic Gram-positive rod. It can cause gangrene in contaminated wounds due to its ability to produce haemolysin. The neurotoxic effect is produced by tetenospasmin. Vaccination is usually repeated every 10 years.

14. The following are contraindications to spinal anaesthesia
A, C, D, E
Local and systemic infections are contraindications to spinal and epidural techniques, as are neurological conditions such as MS.
There is a high risk of catastrophic hypotension in shocked patients.

15. The nerves most commonly injured during patient handling in theatre include
B, C, E

16. Abdominal wound dehiscence
B, C, D
Serosanguinous discharge heralds dehiscence, which usually occurs 5–10 days postoperatively. There are many risk factors that will precipitate this condition. These can be divided into general factors relating to premorbid medical and nutritional status and local factors relating to tissue characteristics.
Jenkins' rule dictates that the suture material should be at least four times longer than the wound.

17. The following are used to assess fluid status
A, C, E
Changes in haematocrit, in the absence of bleeding and serum electrolytes, urea and creatinine, are useful indicators of fluid status.

18. The following blood products are derived from more than one donor
A, E, F
Platelets can be prepared from single or pooled donations. Immunoglobulins are also pooled.

19. Obesity in surgical patients is associated with the following
A, B, C, E
Other complications result from difficulty in performing surgery and the presence of associated medical complication such as cardiovascular disease and diabetes.

20. The following clotting factors are vitamin K dependent
A, D, F, G
The coagulation-inhibiting proteins C and S are also vitamin K dependent.

21. Venous anatomy
A, B, E
The azygos drains into the SVC. The IVC has a short intrathoracic course before entering the right atrium.

22. Smokers have increased risk of postoperative pneumonia due to
A, B, D
Although obesity and inability to cough are independent risk factors, they are not increased in smokers.

23. Surgical trauma has the following metabolic effects
A, C, D, E
Trauma has a diabetogenic effect leading to hyperglycaemia.

24. Type IV or delayed hypersensitivity
A, B, E
Rheumatoid arthritis is immune complex mediated or type III. Cell-mediated hypersensitivity is slow, occurring over a 24–48 hour period.

25. The following protective clothing is mandatory for a trauma team member
A, D, E

26. Regarding disseminated intravascular coagulation
A, C, E
Fibrinogen levels are low with elevation of fibrin degradation products in DIC. Treatment is aimed at the primary pathology and supporting the patient with blood products.

27. The following are features of cardiac tamponade
A, B, E
The elevated JVP is not always present as the patient may be hypovolaemic. Kussmaul's sign is elevated JVP on inspiration. Beck's triad is muffled heart sounds, hypotension and distended neck veins.

28. Regarding the traumatized child
A only
Unlike adults, children are usually given colloids rather than crystalloid. Significant intrathoracic and intra-abdominal injuries can be sustained without any external clues. In those cases requiring investigation for suspicion of visceral damage, CT is the modality of choice in the stable patient.

29. A fracture through the angle of the mandible displaces
C, D, E
This is a result of the pull of masseter and medial pterygoid.

30. Anatomy of the heart
A, E, F
The left coronary artery has two main branches: the left anterior descending and the circumflex artery. The posterior descending (interventricular) artery is a branch of the right coronary. Most of the cardiac venous blood drains into the cardiac veins and the right atrium ultimately.

31. Recognised indications for emergency laparotomy in a trauma patient
A, B, C, D
Although this raises suspicion of splenic trauma, further assessment is indicated if the patient is stable.

32. Valsalva manoeuvre
A, C, D, E
Remember that CO = Sv × HR and BP = CO × SVR (CO, cardiac output; Sv, stroke volume; HR, heart rate; BP, blood pressure; SVR, systemic vascular resistance). The increased intrathoracic pressure generated by the manoeuvre reduces venous return. This in turn reduces stroke volume and hence CO. The SVR rises (vasoconstriction) to maintain a constant BP. After the termination of the manoeuvre there is a sudden increase in Sv, but BP has to remain constant. This is achieved by reducing SVR, HR or both. Change in HR is achievable more quickly and the patient develops reflex bradycardia due to increased vagal activity.

33. Phrenic nerves
B, C, D

The ventral rami of C3–C5 give rise to this nerve which descends in the thorax anterior to the lung hila; the right closely related to the great veins and the left to the great arteries.

34. In the cardiac cycle
A, B, D

The QRS complex corresponds with the 1st heart sound. The 'v' wave of the jugular vein corresponds with ventricular systole and its excessive enlargement is associated with tricuspid regurgitation.

35. Methods of delivering 100% inspired oxygen to patients
B, C, D

Another way of delivering a very high O_2 concentration is a tightly fitting mask and a reservoir bag.

36. Hepatic encephalopathy
A, C, E

Large protein load or blood in gastrointestinal tract will precipitate encephalopathy in susceptible patients.

37. Typical features of a malignant neoplasm
A, C, D

Cancer cells show variation in size with a high nucleus:cytoplasm ratio. The nuclei tend to be hyperchromatic and exhibit abnormal mitoses.

38. The following factors enhance angiogenesis of metastases
A, B, D

Other factors include basic fibroblast growth factor. Angiostatin and transforming growth factor β inhibit angiogenesis.

39. Fat necrosis of the breast
A, C

This usually occurs in middle-aged and older women with clinical signs that may be identical to carcinoma. A history of trauma is not sufficient to make the diagnosis as trauma to the breast may bring a carcinoma to the patient's attention.

40. Neurofibromatosis
A, B, D

Neurofibromatosis usually presents in adult life. There is a 3% risk of malignant transformation.

41. Brain tumours
B, D, E

Brain tumours account for about 2% of deaths in the West.

The commonest tumour in childhood is medulloblastoma of the cerebellar vermis. Supratentorial tumours increase in incidence after adolescence.

42. Bilirubin
D, E

Bilirubin is a metabolite of haemoglobin and other haem-containing proteins. Unconjugated bilirubin is not water soluble and is linked to albumin in the plasma. In the hepatocyte bilirubin is conjugated and excreted in the bile. Bacterial action in the gut converts bilirubin to urobilinogen. Some of the urobilinogen is then absorbed and recycled or excreted in the urine.

Cholesterol is a precursor for bile salts of which deoxycholic acid is one.

43. The following are recognised urachal abnormalities
A, B, C, D

44. Carcinoma of the gall bladder
A, C

The condition is three times more common in females than males and may present with jaundice due to hepatic duct or liver involvement. Surgically treated patients have a quoted 5-year survival of about 16% whereas those treated conservatively have a survival rate of 4%.

45. Indications for preoperative chest X-ray (CXR) include
A, C, D, E

Any patient with symptoms and/or signs of acute or chronic cardiopulmonary disease should have a preoperative CXR. Patients undergoing cardiac or thoracic operations and those having operations for tumours that may metastasize to the lungs should also have a CXR.

46. The following are common indications for inserting a central venous catheter
B, D, E

Other indications include assessment of CO using a pulmonary artery flotation catheter and for infusing parenteral nutrition. Central venous lines are relatively long and have a small diameter. Both of these factors reduce the flow rate through a catheter making them less than ideal for infusing large volumes of fluid in a short period of time.

47. Long-term dialysis is associated with
B, C, D, E

48. Pneumatic anti-shock garments
B, C, D

The garment is not used to cover the thorax nor in cases of diaphragmatic rupture as the increased intra-abdominal pressure will cause respiratory embarrassment.

49. Lung compliance
All true
Compliance of any hollow viscus is a measure of change in volume per change in transmural pressure, i.e. compliance $= \Delta V / \Delta P$.

50. Regarding intracranial pressure (ICP)
A, B, C, E, F
Cerebral perfusion pressure $=$ Systemic blood pressure $-$ ICP
Increased ICP produces hypertension and bradycardia – the so-called Cushing's response.

EMQs

Theme: Skin lesions
61-e

62-a This is a strawberry naevus or cavernous angioma. They usually regress spontaneously without leaving a scar.

63-d This is a melanoma unless proven otherwise on histology. Urgent excision biopsy is required.

64-c This is a typical history of these benign lesions which regress spontaneously after 1–3 months.

Theme: Anaemia
65-b This condition is inherited as an autosomal dominant mostly in northern Europeans. The defect is in the cell membrane which leads to premature cell destruction.

66-e The ESR is low because of the inability of sickle cells to form rouleaux. The definitive diagnosis is made on Hb electrophoresis.

67-c

Theme: Prophylactic antibiotics
68-a Cover against skin organisms is required, therefore flucloxacillin can also be used.

69-h Wide spectrum and anti-anaerobic cover is needed here. Cefuroxime may be substituted by gentamicin and amoxycillin.

70-f Amoxycillin and gentamicin is an alternative.

Theme: Fluid replacement in 24 hours
71-g This patient needs a daily maintenance of 2.5–3 l. In addition to this, NGT losses are replaced with equal volumes of normal saline. Potassium is corrected as needed.

72-c The apparent hyponatraemia is dilutional. Fluid restriction, low sodium intake and a combination of diuretics are usually employed to shed the excess fluid.

73-h Again, gastrointestinal losses are replaced with 0.9% saline. Attention needs to be paid to potassium requirement.

Theme: Chest pain

74-f The history can be confusing but this condition should be suspected in the absence of cardiac pathology on further investigations. Oesophageal manometry is used to make the diagnosis.

75-b

76-d Tietze's syndrome or costochondritis presents as pain and swelling over the sternocostal junction. This is usually evident on palpation.

Theme: Blood transfusion

77-g This female is of child-bearing age and should receive O RhD negative blood if B RhD negative is not available to prevent the risk of haemolytic disease of the newborn in the future.

78-e Although this patient can receive A, B, O and AB red blood cells, i.e. they are a universal recipient, they can only accept serum from AB RhD positive.

79-c The development of anti-RhD antibodies does not carry the grave consequences that it does in females of child-bearing age.

Theme: Glasgow Coma Scale (GCS)

80-g $E = 3, M = 4, V = 4$

81-f $E = 2, M = 5, V = 3$

82-a $E = 1, M = 2, V = 2$

Theme: Haemorrhagic shock

83-c He has lost between 800 and 1500 ml of blood. Note the narrow pulse pressure.

84-e Her pulse is likely to be fast and thready and her BP will have started to decrease.

85-f The blood loss is likely to be well over 2 l.

There are only four classes of shock in common use, numbered I–IV.

Theme: The inflamed or swollen breast

86-b This may later develop into a breast abscess.

87-g This is treated by aspiration and suppressing lactation.

88-e The age and the hard mass point to this diagnosis.

Theme: Management of abdominal trauma

89-d This patient appears relatively stable and if the peritoneum is intact he may be observed.

90-b She is stable enough to undergo DPL but not to be transported to the CT scanner.

91-a Gunshot wound is an indication for laparotomy even if the patient was not shocked.

Theme: Lumps and bumps

92-b A dermoid cyst is a subcutaneous lump that develops mostly in the midline and along lines of fusion in the face and neck. It results from inclusion of epidermal cells deeper to the skin either as a congenital anomaly or secondary to trauma.

93-d This is a benign lump which results from an osteoma of the outer table of the skull.

94-c This is also known as dermatofibroma.

Theme: Causes of reduced urine output

95-g The urinary sodium in prerenal renal failure is usually less than 20 mmol/l.

96-d Hypotensive episodes during cardiac surgery may precipitate renal failure.

Theme: Management of intestinal polyps

97-e It is not possible to establish adequate clearance distally and preserve the anal sphincter. The whole of the colon has to be excised to avoid the risk of developing malignancy elsewhere.

98-d These polyps do not have a malignant potential and can be left alone.

99-h This operation involves the excision of the whole of the colon and rectum and an ileoanal anastomosis. It is a complex operation but has the advantage of preserving continence.

Theme: Staging of cancer

100-b Dukes' A is limited to the wall, B extends beyond the wall and C involves mesenteric lymph nodes. Dukes' original classification was for tumours of the rectum alone and did not include a D stage which signifies spread beyond the regional nodes or involvement of adjacent structures.

101-e Clarke's levels are: I, confined to the epidermis; II, extends to papillary dermis; III, extends to papillary/reticular junction; IV, extends into the reticular dermis; and V, tumours invading the subcutaneous tissue.

102-g

Theme: Management of breast conditions

103-g This is the most commonly used form of treatment for stage I and II disease. It is followed by radiotherapy to the breast.

104-e This woman's age precludes any more aggressive form of treatment.

105-d Symptomatic gynaecomastia may require surgical treatment.

PRACTICE PAPER TWO: CORE MODULES

MCQs

1. Cell cycle

A   DNA manufacture occurs during G1 and G2 stages
B   S stage is the resting period preceding cell division
C   Cardiac myocytes exist in G0 at all times
D   Hepatocytes cannot be induced to leave the G0 stage and enter the cycle
E   Competence growth factors can transform cells from G0 to G1

2. Adult respiratory distress syndrome (ARDS)

A   Is associated with massive trauma
B   Is characterized by a rise in the left atrial pressure
C   Is associated with high compliance
D   Is associated with V/Q mismatch
E   The alveolar membrane function is impaired

3. Baroreceptors

A   Are located in the coronary sinus
B   Respond to a rise in blood pressure only
C   A rise in blood pressure increases the length of the cardiac cycle
D   Produce the Bainbridge reflex
E   Their action is mediated by sympathetic and parasympathetic nerves

4. Myocardial contusion

A   Mostly affects the left ventricle
B   Is associated with sternal fractures
C   May predispose to a ventricular aneurysm
D   Presents with a haemothorax
E   Rhythm abnormalities are rare

5. **Immunoglobulins**

A   IgG is composed of a light chain and a heavy chain
B   Are five different classes
C   IgM has a secretory component
D   IgE may be attached to mast cells
E   Are capable of activating the complement cascade

6. **The following are mandatory in monitoring patients under general anaesthesia**

A   ECG
B   Hourly blood gas analysis
C   Pulse oximetry
D   Blood pressure
E   Temperature

7. *Staphylococcus aureus*

A   Causes osteomeylitis
B   Is a Gram-positive coccus
C   Forms golden colonies on culture
D   Is sensitive to benzylpenicillin
E   Produces coagulase

8. **Regarding diabetic patients**

A   An insulin-dependent diabetic will require lesser doses of insulin in the
     immediate postoperative period
B   A non-insulin dependent diabetic on metformin should miss the morning dose on
     the day of surgery
C   They should be placed first on the operating list
D   They have a higher incidence of wound infection
E   An insulin sliding scale is not usually required for NIDDM patients on oral
     hypoglycaemic

9. **Patients with obstructive jaundice**

A   Require broad-spectrum antibiotic prophylaxis preoperatively
B   Have fluid overload and should be maintained on about 1.5 l of 5% dextrose per
     24 hours

C   Should be infused with albumin solution to correct hypoalbuminaemia
D   Coagulopathy should be corrected with fresh frozen plasma infusion
E   Have increased incidence of wound complications

10. The following viruses are associated with carcinogenesis

A   Hepatitis B virus
B   Hepatitis A virus
C   Human papilloma virus
D   Epstein–Barr virus
E   Orthomyxoviruses

11. Regarding keloid

A   It occurs most commonly in black people
B   It is the same as hypertrophic scar
C   It occurs most commonly on the torso
D   It should be treated prophylactically by radiation
E   It rarely recurs if excised early

12. The following nerves are blocked when performing inguinal hernia repair under local anaesthetic

A   The femoral nerve
B   The iliohypogastric nerve
C   The ilioinguinal nerve
D   The lateral cutaneous nerve of the thigh
E   The obturator nerve
F   The genital branch of the genitofemoral nerve

13. Squamous cell carcinoma of the skin

A   Is predisposed to UV light
B   May occur in chronic ulcers
C   Is treated operatively
D   Is slow growing and does not metastasize to lymph nodes
E   Does not respond to radiotherapy

14. Regarding breast abscess

A   Most puerperal abscesses are caused by *Streptococci*
B   It is associated with smoking
C   It should be treated by incision and drainage
D   It is associated with fibroadenoma
E   Non-puerperal abscesses are caused by Gram-negative organisms
F   It may be complicated by mammary duct fistula

15. The following promote wound healing

A   Apocrine cells
B   Macrophages
C   Platelets
D   Erythrocytes
E   Endothelial cells

16. Fluid replacement in a 70 kg man

A   Infusion of 1 l of 0.9% saline increases the ICF by 0.5 l
B   Infusion of 1 l of 5% dextrose increase the intravascular compartment by 0.07 l
C   Infusion of 0.5 l of 0.9% saline increases the ECF by 0.5 l
D   Infusion of 1 l of colloid immediately increases the ICF by 0.2 l
E   Infusion of 1 l of 0.9% saline increases the intravascular compartment by ~ 0.18 l

17. Acid–base balance

A   High base excess represents CO_2 retention
B PaO_2 is equal to FiO_2
C   Base excess is the amount of acid or base needed to correct pH
D   Renal correction of respiratory acidosis is maximal after 10 minutes
E   Base excess is normally 0 ± 2 mmol/l

18. Regarding the clotting cascade

A   Calcium is an important constituent
B   It occurs in acellular serum
C   Defects can be measured using the bleeding time
D   APTT assesses the activity of the intrinsic system
E   The INR is a ratio of the patient's APTT compared to normal

19. **The following are recognised functions of macrophages**

A Production of complement
B Phagocytosis
C Antigen presentation
D Cytokine production
E Production of fibrocartilage

20. **Regarding nutritional requirement**

A A 70 kg man needs 1500 kcal per day
B It increases during periods of surgical stress
C It is best delivered through the enteral route
D About 10 g of protein are needed for an average person per day
E Carbohydrates have the highest energy content per gram

21. **Prostaglandins**

A Produce fever
B Sensitize nociceptive nerve fibres
C Protect the gastric mucosa
D Suppress inflammation
E Inhibit platelet aggregation

22. **Amyloid**

A May be associated with multiple myeloma
B Exists in the cross-beta pleated sheet formation
C May be secondary to scleroderma
D Stains salmon-red with Congo red stain
E Rarely affects the kidneys

23. **The following scoring systems are used to assess trauma patients**

A Injury Severity Score (ISS)
B Glasgow Coma Scale (GCS)
C APACHE II
D International Trauma Score (ITS)
E Revised Trauma Score (RTS)

24. **The following may impair ventilation**

A   Brain trauma
B   Cervical spine transection
C   Flail chest
D   Obstructed airway
E   Intoxication

25. **Blood is routinely withdrawn from a trauma patient for**

A   Coagulation screen
B   Full blood count
C   Drug screen
D   Cross match purposes
E   Arterial blood gases

26. **The following indicate a positive result for diagnostic peritoneal lavage**

A   Increased pain on performing the procedure
B   Aspiration of blood
C   The appearance of the lavage fluid in a chest drain
D   Developing hypotension on introducing the fluid
E   The passage of a large volume of urine on introducing the lavage fluid

27. **Extradural haematoma**

A   Commonly occurs secondary to a venous bleed
B   Develops slowly over a period of a few weeks
C   Is associated with a lucid period
D   Is commonly associated with a skull fracture

28. **Regarding the pregnant trauma patient**

A   Hypocapnoea occurs towards the end of pregnancy
B   Signs of shock appear with smaller blood loss
C   The patient is resuscitated in a tilted position by raising the left hip
D   Fluid replacement should be cautious due to the risk of foetal oedema
E   There is a risk of Rhesus sensitization

29. The pericardium

A Fuses with the central tendon of the diaphragm
B The pericardial cavity lies between the two layers of the serous pericardium
C Is attached to the sternum by sternopericardial ligaments
D Heavy calcification is associated with TB
E Restrictive pericarditis may present with ascites

30. Signs of spinal shock

A Tachycardia
B Hypertension
C Spastic paralysis
D Priapism
E Absent reflexes

31. Pulmonary anatomy

A Each lung is composed of 15 segments
B Venous drainage follows the segmental arrangement
C Bronchial veins contain deoxygenated blood
D An inhaled foreign body is likely to enter the right lung
E The apical segment of the right lower lobe is the most dependent segment in the supine patient

32. The following conditions are dealt with in the primary survey

A Fractured left leg
B Pneumothorax
C GCS of 10
D Small amount of frank blood per urethra
E Profuse bleeding from scalp wound

33. Pleural pressure

A Is negative throughout a normal breathing cycle
B Becomes more negative on inspiration
C Is equal to alveolar pressure at the end of expiration
D Has a positive value on coughing

34. **Conditions that impair gas exchange**

A   Pneumonia
B   Fibrosing alveolitis
C   Pulmonary embolus
D   Asthma
E   Pulmonary oedema

35. **The following methods are used to measure cardiac output**

A   Thermodilution
B   Pulse and blood pressure
C   Echocardiography
D   CT scan
E   Indicator dilution technique

36. **The following are complications of acute renal failure**

A   Hyperkalaemia
B   Hypercalcaemia
C   Pulmonary oedema
D   ARDS
E   Metabolic acidosis

37. **Shock may cause the following gastrointestinal conditions**

A   Hepatitis
B   Pancreatitis
C   Ulcerative colitis
D   Acalculous cholecystitis
E   Stress ulceration

38. **The following muscles participate in respiration**

A   Pectoralis minor
B   External intercostal
C   Rectus abdominis
D   Scalenus anterior
E   Sternocleidomastoid

39. The following cancers are associated with radiation exposure

A   Leukaemia
B   Lung
C   Squamous cell carcinoma of the skin
D   Thyroid
E   Basal cell carcinoma of the skin

40. Bilateral gynaecomastia is associated with

A   Leprosy
B   Prostate cancer
C   Testicular cancer
D   Liver failure
E   Digoxin therapy
F   Klinefelter's syndrome

41. Carcinoma of the breast

A   Is mostly ductal adenocarcinoma
B   Occurs most commonly in the upper outer quadrant
C   Mastectomy has a better survival rate than wide local excision for early cancers
D   Occurs with equal frequency in the two lower quadrants

42. Dissection of the thoracic aorta

A   Occurs more commonly in hypertensive patients
B   Type B is associated with aortic regurgitation
C   Is best diagnosed by arteriography
D   May be managed conservatively
E   Is associated with paraplegia

43. Hepatitis B infection

A   The prevalence of carriers is higher in the Far East than in the West
B   The presence of HBeAg indicates chronicity of the infection
C   The presence of HBeAg indicates infectivity
D   The infection may be subclinical

44. Oesophageal varices

A   Occur because of communication between systemic and portal venous systems
B   Produce haemorrhage in 50% of patients per year
C   May be treated by portocaval shunt
D   May be treated by distal oesophagectomy
E   Haemorrhage may precipitate hepatic encephalopathy

45. Preoperative preparation of the skin

A   Shaving the skin 1 day before surgery reduces the risk of wound infection
B   Chlorhexidine is faster acting than povidone-iodine
C   Chlorhexidine is longer acting than povidone-iodine
D   The use of a scrubbing brush reduces the risk of wound infection
E   Preoperative showering of patient with Hibiscrub reduces the rate of wound infection

46. Laser in surgery

A CO_2 laser is invisible
B   NdYAG is used to treat oesophageal carcinoma
C   Argon is commonly used for cervical lesions
D   NdYAG is green in colour
E   Argon is absorbed by red pigment making it useful in treating retinal disease

47. The following are recognized oncogenes

A   *sis*
B   *ras*
C   *erbB$_2$*
D   *p53*
E   *myc*

48. The following factors adversely affect the accuracy of pulse oximetry

A   The level of carbon dioxide bound to haemoglobin
B   Nail varnish
C   Shivering
D   Ambient light
E   Depth of anaesthesia

49. Acute haemolytic reaction following blood transfusion

A   Occurs in 90% of mismatched transfusions
B   Usually leads to haemolysis of recipient red blood cells
C   Is due to Rhesus incompatiblity in most cases
D   Presents with chest and lumbar pain
E   Carries a risk of developing acute renal failure

50. Tension pneumothorax

A   The mediastinum shifts to the affected side
B   Can occur with open pneumothorax
C   Untreated, the patient may die because of hypoxia
D   The breath sounds are absent on the affected side
E   The JVP is elevated

EMQs

Theme: Management of an obstructed airway in trauma

Options:
a   15 l of oxygen through face mask
b   10 l of oxygen through face mask and reservoir bag
c   Guedel airway
d   Oropharyngeal airway
e   Nasopharyngeal airway
f   Cricothyroidotomy
g   Endotracheal intubation

For each of the case scenarios below, choose the single most likely option from the list above. Each option may be used once, more than once or not at all.

61. An unconscious patient presents with a positive gag reflex.
62. An unconscious patient presents with a negative gag reflex.
63. A conscious patient presents with severe orofacial trauma and rhinorrhoea.

Theme: Surgical incisions

Options:
a   Upper midline
b   Lower midline
c   Right lateral thoracotomy
d   Left lateral thoracotomy

e   Right subcostal
f   Bilateral subcostal
g   a&c
h   a&d

For each of the case scenarios below, choose the single most likely option from the list above. Each option may be used once, more than once or not at all.

64.   Ivor–Lewis oesophagectomy.
65.   Bilateral adrenalectomy.
66.   Anterior resection of the rectum.

Theme: Correcting coagulation defects

Options:
a   Tranexamic acid
b   Fresh frozen plasma
c   Parenteral vitamin K
d   Factor VIII
e   Fresh frozen plasma, platelets and tranexamic acid
f   Platelets and tranexamic acid
g   Enteral vitamin K

For each of the case scenarios below, choose the single most likely option from the list above. Each option may be used once, more than once or not at all.

67.   An elderly man is known to have AF and is on warfarin. He presents to A&E with epistaxis. His pulse is 120 bpm and BP is 100/65 mmHg. The INR is 5.
68.   A patient presents with obstructive jaundice secondary to carcinoma of the pancreas. His INR is 1.9 and he is due to have ERCP and stenting next week.
69.   You are called to see a patient in ITU 4 hours post laparotomy for faecal peritonitis. He is bleeding from the wound and oozing into the abdominal drain. Recent blood tests show an INR of 3 and elevated fibrin degradation products.

Theme: Anaesthesia

Options:
a   General anaesthesia
b   Epidural and sedation
c   Local infiltration and sedation
d   Bier's block
e   Local anaesthetic field block
f   Paravertebral block
g   Brachial plexus block

For each of the case scenarios below, choose the single most likely option from the list above. Each option may be used once, more than once or not at all.

70. An 81-year-old man presents with severe knee pain secondary to osteoarthritis. He has mild angina and severe emphysema and is to undergo a total knee replacement.
71. A 64-year-old man is admitted with peritonitis secondary to a perforated viscus. He had a myocardial infarct 3 months ago.
72. An elderly woman presents with a severely displaced Colles' fracture.

Theme: Complications of blood transfusion

Options:
a   Immediate haemolytic reaction
b   Febrile reaction
c   Allergic reaction
d   Chilling
e   Septicaemia
f   Delayed haemolytic reaction
g   Viral hepatitis

For each of the case scenarios below, choose the single most likely option from the list above. Each option may be used once, more than once or not at all.

73. A patient develops a temperature of 38°C and headache 3 hours after the start of a blood transfusion.
74. A 65-year-old woman presents 1 week post transfusion with jaundice, anaemia and fever.
75. A patient is transfused with blood for acute gastrointestinal bleeding. Half an hour after the beginning of transfusion he develops a temperature of 39.5°C, tachycardia and hypotension. There is no evidence of haemolysis.

Theme: Oxygen therapy

Options:
a   28% maximum via face mask
b   35% via face mask
c   10 l/min of oxygen through face mask and reservoir bag
d   CPAP
e   IPPV
f   Room air
g   IPPV with 50 cm H_2O of PEEP

For each of the case scenarios below, choose the single most likely option from the list above. Each option may be used once, more than once or not at all.

76. A young man is admitted with respiratory embarrassment secondary to flail chest.
77. A patient develops mild respiratory acidosis and hypoxia following oesophagectomy. The CXR shows severe atelectasis.

78. A 45-year-old patient is brought into A&E having sustained a road traffic accident. He is in haemorrhagic shock but the airway is patent and there is no thoracic trauma.

Theme: The unconscious adult

Options:

a   Alcohol intoxication
b   Extradural haematoma
c   Subdural haematoma
d   Hypoglycaemia
e   Opiate overdose
f   Diffuse axonal injury
g   Intracerebral haemorrhage

For each of the case scenarios below, choose the single most likely option from the list above. Each option may be used once, more than once or not at all.

79. A 35-year-old wicket keeper hit on the head with a ball. He lost consciousness for 2 minutes but recovered afterwards. Three hours later he is brought to hospital unconscious.
80. A young, unkempt man is brought to hospital. He is unconscious and has a low respiratory rate. There are no signs of trauma but his pupils are constricted.
81. An elderly woman sustains a head injury following a fall on her right side. On examination she has left hemiparesis and extensive bruising on the right side of her head.

Theme: Classification of fractures

Options:

a   Transverse
b   Spiral
c   Pathological
d   Stress
e   Comminuted
f   Open
g   Incomplete

For each of the case scenarios below, choose the single most likely option from the list above. Each option may be used once, more than once or not at all.

82. A 73-year-old female presents with a painful right tibia. The X-ray shows abnormal cortical thickening in a bowed tibia with a visible fracture.
83. A young boy sustained a fall while playing. He has an abrasion over the site of tenderness and the X-ray shows a fracture through one of the cortices.
84. A soldier presents with a fractured metatarsal. There is no history of trauma.

Theme: Causes of shock

Options:

a   Hypovolaemic
b   Cardiogenic
c   Tension pneumothorax
d   Anaphylactic
e   Tamponade
f   Septic

For each of the case scenarios below, choose the single most likely option from the list above. Each option may be used once, more than once or not at all.

85.   Cardiac output 7 l/min, JVP 2 mmHg, SVR 9 Wood units after urinary catheterization for acute retention.
86.   Cardiac output 2 l/min, JVP 25 mmHg, SVR 25 Wood units following myocardial infarction.
87.   Cardiac output 3 l/min, JVP 3 mmHg, SVR 20 Wood units.

Theme: Urgent management of gallstone complications

Options:
a   Cholecystectomy
b   Common bile duct exploration
c   ERCP and stone extraction
d   Analgesia
e   c&g
f   Pancreatoduodenectomy
g   Antibiotics

For each of the case scenarios below, choose the single most likely option from the list above. Each option may be used once, more than once or not at all.

88.   A patient with known gallstones presents with right upper quadrant pain and vomiting. Her temperature is 36.8°C and WBC is normal.
89.   A patient with cholecystitis develops a palpable gall bladder and swinging pyrexia despite antibiotic treatment.
90.   A patient who is awaiting cholecystectomy presents with acute abdominal pain, fever and jaundice. Her temperature is 38.5°C, WBC 21×10^9 per ml, bilirubin 75 μmol/l and amylase 1255 iu/ml.

Theme: Management of postoperative complications of cardiac surgery

Options:
a   Intra-aortic balloon pump counterpulsation
b   0.18% saline infusion

c   Potassium supplement
d   Amiodorone
e   ACE inhibitors
f   Lignocaine
g   Pacemaker

For each of the case scenarios below, choose the single most likely option from the list above. Each option may be used once, more than once or not at all.

91. A patient develops a fast and irregular heart rhythm but the blood pressure is normal. The ECG reveals no P waves and irregular QRS complexes. Serum chemistry reveals the following: Na 128 mmol/l, K 3.3 mmol/l, Mg 0.9 mmol/l.
92. A patient develops bradycardia of 40 bpm and mild hypotension with marked decrease in the urine output.
93. A patient with poor cardiac output does not respond adequately to inotropes following quadruple bypass. The preoperative ejection fraction is 30%.

Theme: Staging of breast cancer

Options:
a   Manchester 0
b   Manchester TIS
c   Manchester I
d   Manchester II
e   Manchester IIIa
f   Manchester IIIb
g   Manchester IV
h   Manchester V

For each of the case scenarios below, choose the single most likely option from the list above. Each option may be used once, more than once or not at all.

94. Tumour size (T) = 1.5 cm. No palpable lymph nodes.
95. Tumour size (T) = 3.2 cm. Mobile axillary lymph node.
96. Fungating tumour. Bone metastasis.

Theme: Treatment of benign breast conditions

Options:
a   Gamolenic acid
b   Glimpepiride
c   Tamoxifen
d   Reassurance
e   Wide excision
f   Needle biopsy
g   Microdochectomy

For each of the case scenarios below, choose the single most likely option from the list above. Each option may be used once, more than once or not at all.

97. A 25-year-old woman complains of severe breast pain which is worst preceding menstruation. She has not had any treatment for the pain.

98. A woman in her fifties, with persistent green discharge from a single breast duct, is diagnosed with ductal ectasia. She finds her symptoms distressing.

99. A 21-year-old woman presents with a painless breast lump. She has a fibroadenoma both clinically and on USS.

Theme: Palliative management of advanced cancer

Options:

a   Skeletal traction
b   Radiotherapy
c   Nerve block
d   Chemotherapy
e   Internal fixation
f   External fixation
g   Surgical resection

For each of the case scenarios below, choose the single most likely option from the list above. Each option may be used once, more than once or not at all.

100. A patient who is known to have pancreatic cancer is suffering from severe back pain which is not responding to very large doses of opiates.

101. An elderly man with known prostatic cancer presents with pathological fracture of the femoral neck.

102. A woman presents 7 years following mastectomy with severe thoracic wall pain. X-rays and bone scan show metastases.

Theme: Acid-base balance

Options:

a   Metabolic alkalosis
b   Metabolic acidosis
c   Uncompensated respiratory alkalosis
d   Uncompensated respiratory acidosis
e   Compensated respiratory alkalosis
f   Compensated respiratory acidosis

For each of the case scenarios below, choose the single most likely option from the list above. Each option may be used once, more than once or not at all.

103. pH 7.3, PaO_2 8.5 kPa, $PaCO_2$ 9.8 kPa, HCO_3 33 mmol/l.
104. pH 7.55, PaO_2 10 kPa, $PaCO_2$ 7.3 kPa, HCO_3 43 mmol/l.
105. pH 7.3, PaO_2 8.5 kPa, $PaCO_2$ 8.0 kPa, HCO_3 27 mmol/l.

ANSWERS TO PRACTICE PAPER TWO

The letters of the correct answers are given

MCQs

1. Cell cycle
C, E

Cells are divided into labile, stable and permanent. Labile cells are dividing all the time (such as the cells of mucous membranes) whereas stable cells are not dividing but have the potential to do so (such as hepatic and renal cells). Permanent cells always exist in G0 and cannot join the cell cycle (e.g. nerve and muscle cells).

The cell cycle is composed of 'G1' (first gap) stage, 'S' (synthesis) stage when DNA is manufactured, 'G2' (second gap) followed finally by 'M' (mitosis) stage. The cell then enters G1 stage if it is labile in order to undergo another cycle. The 'G0' stage is outside the cell cycle and a stable but not a permanent cell can be induced to leave it and enter the cycle (at G1) by a competence factor. Progression factors stimulate DNA synthesis in competent cells (i.e. those in the cycle).

2. Adult respiratory distress syndrome (ARDS)
A, D, E

In ARDS there is reduced compliance and impaired membrane function due to oedema and fibrosis as the disease process progresses.

3. Baroreceptors
C, E

These are located in the carotid sinuses and the aortic arch. They respond to changes in blood pressure by modulating autonomic effects on the heart so as to reduce heart rate in hypertension and *vice versa*.

4. Myocardial contusion
B, C, E

The right ventricle is the most commonly injured heart chamber, be it blunt or penetrating stab injury, by virtue of its anatomical position. Contusion of the myocardium predisposes to the same complications as infarction.

5. Immunoglobulins
B, D, E

Immunoglobulins have a basic structure of two light chains and two heavy chains. The heaviest is IgM being composed of five basic units. IgA is composed of two units linked by a secretory piece.

6. The following are mandatory in monitoring patients under general anaesthesia
A, C, D
Others include capnography and airway pressure.

7. *Staphylococcus aureus*
A, B, C, E
Flucloxacillin is the penicillin most commonly used to treat this group of bacteria (except the methicillin-resistant strains).

8. Regarding diabetic patients
B, C, D, E
All patients have an increased requirement for insulin postoperatively. This is part of the inflammatory response to surgery. Most NIDDM patients can be managed adequately by missing the morning dose of their oral hypoglycaemic medication. A sliding scale need not be started unless the glucose is $> 12\,mmol/l$.

9. Patients with obstructive jaundice
A, E
Patients with obstructive jaundice may develop renal failure, therefore hydration and strict fluid management to maintain a good urinary output are essential in managing these patients. Hypoalbuminaemia is treated by addressing the underlying pathology and good nutritional support. Coagulopathy is secondary to vitamin K malabsorption and early anticipation of the problem and supplementation should prevent the need for fresh frozen plasma except in emergencies.

10. The following viruses are associated with carcinogenesis
A, C, D
Hepatitis A is not associated with malignancy. Orthomyxoviruses cause respiratory tract infections.

11. Regarding keloid
A, C
Keloid spreads beyond the site of injury, unlike hypertrophic scarring which does not. Excision of keloid is often complicated by recurrence and radiation has not been shown to affect the outcome. Some advocate the use of intradermal injection of steroid with a variable effect.

12. The following nerves are blocked when performing inguinal hernia repair under local anaesthetic
B, C, F

13. Squamous cell carcinoma of the skin
A, B, C
Squamous cell carcinoma is faster growing and has more potential for metastasis than basal cell carcinoma. Poorly differentiated tumours or those in elderly patients may be treated with radiotherapy.

14. Regarding breast abscess
B, F

Staphylococci account for the majority of cases, but anaerobic *Streptococci* and *Bacteroides* can also be responsible. Breast abscesses may be treated with antibiotics and ultrasound-guided needle aspiration.

15. The following promote wound healing
B, C, E

Other cells include neutrophils and myofibroblasts.

16. Fluid replacement in a 70 kg man
B, E

In a 70 kg man the ICF = $\sim$251 and the ECF = $\sim$171. The intravascular fluid compartment which is part of the ECF contains $\sim$31 of water. Normal (0.9%) saline contributes to the ECF only, of which $\sim$18% remains in the intravascular compartment. 5% dextrose contributes to all compartments equally, therefore the intravascular compartment receives only 0.07% of the volume.

17. Acid–base balance
C, E

There is a gradient of about 10 kPa between the inspired/alveolar oxygen partial pressure and the arterial oxygen partial pressure in the normal subject.
The renal response to acid–base disturbance is delayed, occurring over hours to days.

18. Regarding the clotting cascade
A, D

Serum differs from plasma in that it does not contain fibrinogen and therefore will not form a clot. APTT, PT and INR (a ratio of PT) are used to assess the coagulation cascade, whereas platelet function is measured using the bleeding time.

19. The following are recognized functions of macrophages
A, B, C, D

Other functions include production of growth factors necessary for healing, and free radicals and enzymes used in the destruction of bacteria.

20. Regarding nutritional requirement
B, C

Energy requirement is about 40 kcal per kg and the protein requirement is 1.5 g per kg per day.

21. Prostaglandins
A, C, D

Prostaglandins are mediators of inflammation and reducing their production relieves pain, fever and inflammation. Prostacyclins inhibit platelet aggregation and cause vasodilatation.

22. Amyloid
A, B, C, D
The kidneys are frequently affected as well as the spleen, liver and heart.

23. The following scoring systems are used to assess trauma patients
A, B, E
Trauma Score and Injury Severity Score (TRISS) is another scoring system. It incorporates ISS, RTS, age and mechanism of injury. APACHE II (Acute Physiology and Chronic Health Evaluation) is used to score patients in non-trauma situations.

24. The following may impair ventilation
All true
Brain trauma and intoxication affect the ventilatory centre. Spinal transection, at this level, denervates respiratory muscles.

25. Blood is routinely withdrawn from a trauma patient for
B, D, E
Plasma urea and electrolytes are also measured routinely.

26. The following indicate a positive result for diagnostic peritoneal lavage
B, C, E
Passage of large amounts of fluid into a urinary catheter should alert the surgeon who is performing DPL that this is lavage fluid and not urine. If that is the case laparotomy is indicated.

27. Extradural haematoma
C, D
Extradural haematoma occurs commonly after arterial injury especially of the middle meningeal artery. A lucid period intervenes in up to a third of cases but otherwise the presentation is acute.

28. Regarding the pregnant trauma patient
A, E
Pregnancy increases the circulating blood volume by about 50% which results in significant blood loss before the patient exhibits signs of shock. Moreover, foetal shock occurs earlier than maternal shock necessitating aggressive fluid resuscitation.

29. The pericardium
All true
Restrictive pericarditis, as occurs in TB infection resulting in severe calcification, presents with low-output cardiac failure, oedema, ascites and hepatic dysfunction.

30. Signs of spinal shock
D, E
In spinal shock there is hypotension and bradycardia. A cervical or thoracic lesion produces abdominal breathing as other muscles of respiration are paralysed. The paralysis is flaccid in type.

31. Pulmonary anatomy
C, D, E
The lungs are composed of 10 segments each. Each segment is supplied by a segmental bronchus and artery, but the veins tend to drain adjacent segments.

32. The following conditions are dealt with in the primary survey
B, E
The primary survey is mainly concerned with the Airway, Breathing and Circulation. Quick assessment of neurological Dysfunction is made at this stage but therapeutic measures are aimed at life-threatening conditions.

33. Pleural pressure
A, B, D
The alveolar pressure is equal to the atmospheric pressure as long as the glottis is open.

34. Conditions that impair gas exchange
A, B, C, E
Gas exchange is reduced in the presence of any ventilation/perfusion mismatch or if the pathological process affects the exchange membrane.

35. The following methods are used to measure cardiac output
A, C, E
A and E require insertion of a pulmonary artery catheter, whereas echocardiography is non-invasive. The measurements needed to calculate cardiac output are stroke volume and heart rate.

36. The following are complications of acute renal failure
A, C, E
Other complications of acute renal failure include hypocalcaemia, DIC, arrhythmias and reduced immunity.

37. Shock may cause the following gastrointestinal conditions
A, B, D, E
Small and large bowel ischaemia also occur.

38. The following muscles participate in respiration
All true

39. The following cancers are associated with radiation exposure
All true

40. Bilateral gynaecomastia is associated with
All true

41. Carcinoma of the breast
A, B
Mastectomy and wide local excision have the same long-term survival, although the local recurrence rate is higher with the latter. Nearly twice as many carcinomas occur in the outer lower quadrant than the inner lower quadrant.

42. Dissection of the thoracic aorta
A, C, D, E
Type A aneurysm involves the ascending aorta and demands surgical repair, whereas type B is distal, does not involve the aortic valve and can be managed conservatively.

43. Hepatitis B infection
All true

44. Oesophageal varices
A, C, E
The risk of haemorrhage in patients with varices is about 30% in 2 years. Injection sclerotherapy is the treatment of choice for the majority of cases. Oesophagogastric disconnection or gastric transection is occasionally used.

45. Preoperative preparation of the skin
C, E
Shaving produces skin abrasions which results in a higher rate of wound infection if performed a long time before the operation.

46. Laser in surgery
A, B, E
NdYAG is invisible. Cervical lesions are usually treated with CO_2 laser.

47. The following are recognized oncogenes
A, B, C, E
p53 is a tumour suppressor gene.

48. The following factors adversely affect the accuracy of pulse oximetry
B, C, D
Other factors include the presence of methaemoglobin, jaundice, low cardiac output and peripheral vasoconstriction.

49. Acute haemolytic reaction following blood transfusion
D, E
Acute haemolytic reactions are due to ABO incompatibility in most cases. The patient has preformed antibodies to the donor's red blood cells leading to haemolysis of the donated cells. Occasionally, the patient's own cells are haemolysed. Only 1 in 3 mismatched transfusions result in haemolysis because of the fact that group AB accepts all groups and groups A and B accept group O.

50. Tension pneumothorax
D, E

Tension pneumothorax occurs when a one-way valve develops and air collects in the pleural space under pressure. As a result, the mediastinum shifts away from the affected side and the venous return is obstructed resulting in distended neck veins. If left untreated the venous return is progressively diminished until the cardiac output is no longer compatible with life.

EMQs

Theme: Management of an obstructed airway in trauma
61-e This patient may also be managed by chin lift or jaw thrust. There is a risk of vomiting and aspiration if an airway is inserted into the mouth.

62-g This secures the airway and protects it from aspiration.

63-f

Theme: Surgical incisions
64-g

65-f A transverse upper abdominal incision may also be employed.

66-b

Theme: Correcting coagulation defects
67-b This patient is in shock and needs urgent resuscitation and correction of the coagulopathy.

68-c

69-e This is DIC.

Theme: Anaesthesia
70-b This technique will avoid problems weaning him off the ventilator.

71-a The operation is life saving. His recent myocardial infarct puts him at risk of further infarct but there is no choice except general anaesthesia.

72-d This is more effective than local infiltration or 'haematoma block'.

Theme: Complications of blood transfusion
73-b These usually occur secondary to leucocyte antigens and can be treated with antihistamines and antipyretics.

74-f The patient is usually immunized to the antigen at previous transfusion but the concentration of antibodies is too low to manifest as an immediate reaction. Production of further IgG, usually a week later, leads to delayed haemolysis.

75-e The risk is highest in old blood maintained in suboptimal condition or kept out of the refrigerator for too long before transfusion.

Theme: Oxygen therapy

76-e This will treat his flail chest.

77-d Early administration of CPAP on a high dependency unit will prevent deterioration of atelectasis and hopefully avert admission to the ITU.

78-c This will improve the oxygen delivery to tissues.

Theme: The unconscious adult

79-b Extradural haematoma is commonly associated with a skull fracture and classically, but not always, presents with a history of a 'lucid period'.

80-e

81-c Elderly patients are more likely to have a subdural than an extradural haematoma because of brain atrophy and the fact that the dura is adherent to the skull.

Theme: Classification of fractures

82-c This woman is likely to have Paget's disease.

83-g This is an incomplete or greenstick fracture.

84-d This is known as a 'march' fracture.

Theme: Causes of shock

85-f Wood units are derived from the fact that SVR = ΔBP/CO. Therefore, normal SVR is about 15 Wood units. Multiply Wood units by 80 to calculate SVR in dynes sec cm^{-5}. This patient has increased CO in the face of reduced SVR which occurs in sepsis and anaphylaxis, but the history of instrumentation makes sepsis more likely.

86-b A similar picture occurs in tamponade.

87-a

Theme: Urgent management of gallstone complications

88-d This is biliary colic. Antibiotic treatment is not indicated unless there is evidence of sepsis.

89-a Empyema of the gall bladder requires urgent cholecystectomy.

90-e This patient has pancreatitis and cholangitis. Antibiotics, fluid resuscitation and urgent ERCP to decompress the biliary tree are mandatory.

Theme: Management of postoperative complications of cardiac surgery

91-c Atrial fibrillation is the commonest arrhythmia following cardiac surgery and is usually managed by correcting potassium and magnesium levels. Antiarrhythmic agents such as amiodorone are employed if this measure fails, with DC shock being reserved for resistant cases or urgent rhythm conversion.

92-g This patient needs a temporary pacing wire followed by a permanent pacemaker.

93-a This device inflates in diastole and deflates in systole, therefore helps the failing heart by reducing the afterload.

Theme: Staging of breast cancer

94-c T $< 2\,cm$, N_0, M_0 = stage I.

95-d T = 2–$5\,cm$, N_1, M_0 = stage II.

96-g Distant metastasis = stage IV.

Theme: Treatment of benign breast conditions

97-a

98-g

99-d Carcinoma is *very* rare at this age and unless the patient is very concerned a fibroadenoma should be left alone.

Theme: Palliative management of advanced cancer

100-c A coeliac block should help control the pain.

101-e

102-b

Theme: Acid–base balance

103-f The pH shows acidosis which must be respiratory in origin in view of the elevated carbon dioxide. The elevated bicarbonate indicates metabolic alkalosis in an attempt to correct the abnormality. This picture occurs in chronic respiratory disease.

104-a Respiratory compensation occurs within minutes. Here the carbon dioxide rise is an attempt to compensate for the metabolic alkalosis as in pyloric stenosis.

105-d This is similar to question 94 except that the bicarbonate is within normal limits. This occurs in acute ventilatory embarrassment such as in flail chest.

PRACTICE PAPER THREE: CORE MODULES

MCQs

1. The following are tumour suppressor genes

A   Rb (retinoblastoma) gene
B   NF2 neurofibromatosis gene
C   MTS 1
D   *p53*
E   Kirsten *ras* gene

2. Chest radiograph

A   The right heart border is formed by the right ventricle
B   The right heart border is adjacent to the middle lobe of the right lung
C   A haemothorax may easily be missed on a supine film
D   Widening of the mediastinum is associated with dissecting thoracic aneurysm
E   The left atrium is completely invisible on a PA radiograph

3. Pressure measurements in normal heart chambers

A   Right atrium 20 mmHg
B   Right ventricle 20/0 mmHg
C   pulmonary artery 20/6 mmHg
D   left atrium 7 mmHg
E   left ventricle 120/80 mmHg

4. Regarding haemorrhagic shock in an average adult

A   Class I is characterized by loss of 25% of circulating volume
B   There is a slight tachycardia (< 100 bpm) in class I
C   Diastolic blood pressure may rise in class III shock
D   The systolic blood pressure starts to drop after loss of over 2 l of blood
E   Widened pulse pressure is an early signal of significant blood loss
F   Hypotension occurs with smaller blood loss in patients taking β blockers

5. **Regarding haemophilia (A and B)**

A   Factor IX deficiency is called Christmas disease
B   Haemophilia A is due to deficiency of von Willebrand's factor
C   There is prolonged APTT and PT in haemophilia B
D   Both are inherited in an autosomal fashion
E   They are usually treated with fresh frozen plasma

6. **The following variables are used to calculate pH**

A $PaCO_2$
B PaO_2
C   Base excess
D $\log 1/PaCO_2$
E HCO_3^-
F   Base increase

7. **The following are Gram-positive rods**

A   *Escherichia coli*
B   *Clostridium tetani*
C   *Staphylococcus aureus*
D   *Neisseria gonorrhoeae*
E   *Bacillus anthracis*

8. **Regarding surgical patients on long-term steroid therapy**

A   There is an increased risk of wound complications in these patients
B   There is a risk of an Addisonian crisis if their steroids are stopped abruptly
C   There is increased requirement for steroids per- and postoperatively
D   They have a higher risk of peptic ulceration

9. **The following states are associated with compromised immunity**

A   Advanced malignancy
B   Agammaglobulinaemia
C   AIDS
D   Patients on the drug tacrolimus
E   Severe jaundice
F   Chronic renal failure

10. **The following factors increase the risk of wound infection**

A Length of the procedure
B Emergency surgery
C High number of theatre personnel
D Operation on a hollow viscus
E Diabetes

11. **Regarding interosseous needle in children with trauma**

A Only crystalloids can be infused
B The circulation time is about 2 minutes
C The scapula is a common site for placement
D It is preferred to central venous catheter
E Osteomyelitis is a complication

12. **Regarding bowel anastomosis**

A A double layer technique is mandatory
B All layers of the bowel should be included
C A side-to-side bypass may be associated with blind loop syndrome
D An absorbable synthetic material should be used

13. **The following are advantages of epidural over spinal anaesthesia**

A It causes less marked hypotension
B It can be used for postoperative analgesia
C The block is more effective
D It does not affect the sympathetic nerves
E There is less risk of developing headache as a side effect

14. **Regarding diathermy**

A In bipolar diathermy the current passes through the patient's body
B Bipolar diathermy requires a plate of at least $100 \, cm^2$
C Cardiac pacemaker is a relative contraindication
D The frequency of the electric current is 70–150 Hz
E It should be used with care on tissue adjacent to nerves

15. Sterilization by steam

A   Occurs at a higher temperature than dry heat sterilization
B   Does not kill spores
C   Takes a shorter time than dry heat to sterilize instruments
D   Works at subatmospheric pressure
E   Is ideal for sterilizing ointments

16. The intracellular compartment in a 70 kg male

A   Contains about 25 l of water
B   Has a higher osmolality than the intravascular compartment
C   Contains 70% of the body's sodium
D   Is chiefly regulated by hydrostatic pressure
E   Contains 95% of the body's potassium

17. Blunt trauma to the spleen

A   May form a haematoma which displaces the gastric shadow on radiographs
B   Occurs easily in the presence of splenomegaly
C   Is associated with pain that may radiate to the left shoulder
D   Can be treated conservatively
E   Is rare under the age of 12

18. Donated blood is screened for

A   HSV
B   TB
C   HIV
D   Syphilis
E   Hepatitis B virus
F   Hepatitis C virus
G   Gonorrhoea

19. The following are clinical signs of malnutrition

A   Peripheral oedema
B   Angular stomatitis
C   Hypothyroidism
D   Peripheral neuropathy
E   Limb ischaemia
F   Loss of muscle power

20. **The following parameters are set on a PCA syringe driver**

A   Bolus dose
B   Minimum dose per 4 hours
C   Lock-out period
D   Total dose per day
E   Infusion dose during period of sleep

21. **Platelets**

A   Are anucleate
B   Have a life span of about 3 weeks
C   Produce growth factors
D   Have an important role in coagulation
E   Are implicated in TIAs

22. **Metastatic calcification**

A   Occurs in disseminated malignancy
B   Calcium is deposited in normal tissues
C   Is associated with hyperparathyroidism
D   Causes calcification of rheumatic heart valves
E   Occurs with elevated serum calcium
F   Is associated with psammoma bodies

23. **The following disorders are thought to be autoimmune**

A   Systemic lupus erythematosus
B   Hashimoto's thyroiditis
C   Sclerosing cholangitis
D   De Quervain's thyroiditis
E   Scleroderma

24. **Methods of maintaining a patent airway in the traumatized patient**

A   Nasotracheal intubation in mouth trauma and base of skull fracture
B   Jaw thrust
C   Nasopharyngeal airway in the conscious patient
D   Oropharyngeal airway in the conscious patient
E   Tracheostomy

25. Flail chest

A   Is often accompanied by lung contusion
B   Hypoxia is mainly due to hypoventilation
C   Requires ventilation as primary treatment
D   Occurs when two or more ribs are fractured at more than one site
E   Manifests with pulsus paradoxus

26. Methods employed for emergency splintage of a fracture in a patient with multiple trauma

A   Skeletal traction
B   Plaster of Paris
C   Vacuum splints
D   Inflatable jacket splints
E   Traction splints, e.g. Thomas splint

27. The following are recognized complications of burns

A   Renal failure
B   Airway obstruction
C   Acute pancreatitis
D   Inadequate ventilation
E   Haemolysis

28. Cardiac action potential

A   The upstroke of a slow-response action potential is due to Ca^{2+} influx
B   Slow fibres are found in the SA and AV nodes
C   The resting potential is less negative in slow-response fibres
D   The refractory period is longer in fast-response fibres
E   The upstroke of a fast-response action potential is due to Na^+ efflux

29. Surface markings of diaphragmatic openings

A   The opening for the IVC is 1.5 cm right of the midline at the level of the 6th costal cartilage
B   The opening for the aorta is below the transpyloric plane
C   The oesophageal hiatus is in the midline at the level of the 7th costal cartilage
D   The aortic hiatus is to the right of the midline

30. Carcinoma of the bronchus may present with

A   Hypercalcaemia in squamous cell tumours
B   Hoarse voice
C   Cushing's disease in oat cell tumours
D   Horner's syndrome
E   Thrombophlebitis migrans

31. The following layers are encountered on inserting a subclavian venous line

A   Clavipectoral fascia
B   Subclavius
C   Pectoralis minor
D   Pectoralis major
E   Scalenus anterior

32. Indications for dialysis include

A   Rising creatinine
B   Worsening acidosis pH < 7.25
C   Rising urea
D   Fluid overload
E   Pericarditis

33. The following are used to calculate the APACHE score

A   Serum sodium
B   Serum urea
C   Core temperature
D   White cell count
E   GCS
F   Bilirubin

34. The following nerves traverse the diaphragm

A   Vagus
B   Intercostobrachial
C   Hypogastric
D   Greater splanchnic
E   Phrenic

35. The following constitute paraneoplastic syndromes

A Cushing's syndrome in pancreatic carcinoma
B Hypercalcaemia in squamous cell carcinoma of the lung
C Cushing's disease in pituitary adenoma
D Hypoglycaemic attacks secondary to insulinoma
E Hypercalcaemia in metastatic prostate cancer

36. Factors that contribute to development of the adult female breast at puberty

A Testosterone
B Oestradiol
C Insulin growth factor-1
D Growth hormone
E Cortisol
F Prolactin

37. Brain abscess

A Occurs most commonly in the occipital lobe
B The survival rate is better for those presenting with a short history
C Shows up as a ring-enhancing lesion on CT scan
D Is usually primary with no evidence of sepsis elsewhere in the body
E Is not more common in patients with epilepsy

38. The following are recognized eye signs in hyperthyroidism

A Lid lag
B Corneal abrasions
C Cataracts
D Ophthalmoplegia
E Chemosis

39. Hernias around the umbilicus

A In adults are more common in females than males
B May be treated adequately by a truss in adults
C Congenital hernias are common in Africa
D The umbilical cicatrix should be excised at repair
E Should be repaired surgically in infants

40. **The following examinations are necessary before urethral catheterization of a trauma patient**

A Abdominal examination
B Digital rectal examination
C Bowel sounds
D Intravenous urogram
E Look for blood at the external urethral meatus

41. **The following are recognized methods of treating chronic pancreatitis**

A Pancreatoduodenectomy
B Total pancreatectomy
C Stenting of the pancreatic duct
D Lumbar sympathectomy
E Side-to-side pancreatojejunostomy

42. **Blind loop syndrome**

A Is associated with side-to-side bowel anastomoses
B Produces anaemia
C Presents with constipation
D Is associated with accelerated weight gain
E Presents with fever

43. **BRCA1 gene**

A Is associated with sarcoma
B Is inherited in an autosomal fashion
C Is associated with breast cancer
D Is associated with colorectal cancer
E Is associated with ovarian cancer
F Is associated with endometrial cancer

44. **The following organisms cause opportunistic infections**

A *Cryptosporidium* spp.
B *Pneumocystis carinii*
C *Mycobacterium avium-intracellulare*
D *Toxoplasmosis gondii*
E *Candida* spp.

45. **Recognized complications of insertion of a central venous catheter include**

A   Arterial puncture
B   Transient ischaemic attack
C   Cardiac arrhythmia
D   Hepatic abscess
E   Haemothorax

46. **Transfusion with fresh frozen plasma is indicated to correct**

A   INR of 6.5 in a patient who is on warfarin for a prosthetic heart valve
B   An elevated INR in the jaundiced patient
C   Disseminated intravascular coagulation in a septic patient
D   Bleeding from oesophageal varices in a cirrhotic patient
E   Bleeding after cardiopulmonary bypass

47. **Traumatic diaphragmatic rupture**

A   Is more common on the right side
B   Is bilateral in 40% of cases
C   The diagnosis can be made on CXR
D   Is treated conservatively unless hypoxia ensues
E   Presents with surgical emphysema

48. **Base of skull fractures**

A   May be associated with anosmia
B   Rhinorrhoea fluid is positive for glucose on dipstix testing
C   May be complicated by meningitis
D   Of the anterior fossa produces 'panda eyes' sign
E   Skull X-rays are not indicated

49. **Values measured on spirometry**

A   Forced expiratory volume in 1 second
B   Peak expiratory flow rate
C   Total lung capacity
D   Carbon monoxide diffusion test
E   Forced vital capacity

50. The following are useful prognostic factors in breast cancer

A   The oestrogen receptor status
B   Tumour size
C   Nodal status
D   Histological grade
E   Histological type
F   Clinical signs of inflammation

EMQs

Theme: Definition of statistical terms used in medicine

Options:
a   Attributable risk
b   Sensitivity
c   Specificity
d   Relative risk
e   Accuracy
f   Positive predictive value
g   Significance

The following are definitions of statistical terms. Choose the single most likely option from the list above. Each option may be used once, more than once or not at all.

61. A measurement of the ability of the test to give the true result.
62. The ability of a test to identify those who have the disease.
63. A ratio of the disease rate in exposed patients to those unexposed.

Theme: Treatment of obstructive jaundice

Options:
a   Pancreatoduodenectomy
b   Choledochojejunostomy
c   Cholecystojejunostomy and gastrojejunostomy
d   ERCP and stenting
e   ERCP followed by laparoscopic cholecystectomy
f   Open cholecystectomy
g   Open cholecystectomy and intraoperative cholangiogram

For each of the case scenarios below, choose the single most likely option from the list above. Each option may be used once, more than once or not at all.

64. A 75-year-old man presents with progressive jaundice, weight loss and back pain. A CT scan reveals carcinoma of the pancreatic head and coeliac lymphadenopathy.
65. Another patient, aged 63, presents with a history similar to the above, but is found to have a 2.5 cm mass in the pancreatic head with no evidence of spread.
66. A woman in her early forties presents with cholecystitis and jaundice. USS reveals a dilated biliary tree and stones in the common bile duct and gall bladder.

Theme: Immediate management of thoracic trauma

Options:
a   Intercostal drain
b   Pericardiocentesis
c   Needle thoracocentesis
d   Chest radiograph followed by intercostal drain
e   Bilateral intercostal drain
f   Thoracotomy
g   Blood transfusion

For each of the case scenarios below, choose the single most likely option from the list above. Each option may be used once, more than once or not at all.

67. A patient presents with a stab lateral to the sternal edge in the left fifth intercostal space. His pulse is thready and he is hypotensive. There has been no response to 3 l of crystalloids.
68. A woman sustains a fall on her right side. In A&E she has tachypnoea, tachycardia, hypotension and dullness on percussing the right side of her chest.
69. A patient with haemothorax drained 500 ml on inserting an intercostal drain and 100 ml/hour since. The drain has been *in situ* for 2 hours.

Theme: Sterilization and disinfection of surgical instruments

Options:
a   Dry heat autoclave
b   Formaldehyde autoclave
c   Moist heat autoclave
d   Ethylene oxide
e   Glutaraldehyde
f   Gamma radiation
g   Immersion in boiling water

For each of the objects below, choose the single most likely option from the list above. Each option may be used once, more than once or not at all.

70. A stainless steel haemostat
71. Latex gloves
72. Colonoscope
73. Polyglactin suture

Theme: The person capable of giving informed consent

Options:
a   Patient
b   Partner
c   Parents
d   Doctor
e   Psychiatrist
f   Judge
g   Hospital management

For each of the case scenarios below, choose the single most likely option from the list above. Each option may be used once, more than once or not at all.

74.   A 17-year-old patient refuses to have any surgical intervention for suspected appendicitis.
75.   A diabetic patient with chronic stable schizophrenia presents with necrotic ischaemic hallux which requires amputation. He understands the implications but refuses surgery.
76.   A stabbed patient needs an emergency thoracotomy. He is unconscious.

Theme: Nutritional support

Options:
a   Intravenous dextrose
b   Total parenteral nutrition
c   Gastrostomy
d   Jejunostomy
e   Nasojejunal tube
f   High calorie drinks
g   Caecostomy

For each of the case scenarios below, choose the single most likely option from the list above. Each option may be used once, more than once or not at all.

77.   A 65-year-old patient 3 days post partial gastrectomy.
78.   A 21-year-old patient with enterocutaneous fistula following a right hemicolectomy for Crohn's disease.
79.   A patient who is unable to swallow due to a neurological condition.

Theme: Pain relief

Options:
a   Paracetamol
b   Paracetamol and NSAID
c   Weak opiate
d   NSAID and opiate

e   Patient-controlled analgesia
f   Epidural analgesia

For each of the case scenarios below, choose the single most likely option from the list above. Each option may be used once, more than once or not at all.

80. A 70-year-old man who underwent an abdominal aortic aneurysm repair through a transverse abdominal incision.
81. A patient who underwent an inguinal hernia repair.
82. A woman who underwent coronary artery bypass grafting.

Theme: Structures injured during surgery on the neck

Options:
a   Recurrent laryngeal nerve
b   External laryngeal nerve
c   Parathyroid glands
d   Thoracic duct
e   Stellate ganglion
f   Phrenic nerve

For each of the case scenarios below, choose the single most likely option from the list above. Each option may be used once, more than once or not at all.

83. A patient is complaining of tingling in the tips of her fingers.
84. A singer is complaining of her voice becoming weak after singing for a short period of time.
85. A patient presents with unilateral ptosis and small pupil.

Theme: Thoracic trauma

Options:
a   Flail chest
b   Open pneumothorax
c   Tracheal transection
d   Tension pneumothorax
e   Haemothorax
f   Cardiac tamponade
g   Myocardial contusion

For each of the case scenarios below, choose the single most likely option from the list above. Each option may be used once, more than once or not at all.

86. A patient sustained blunt thoracic trauma. On examination the respiratory rate was 30 per minute. The trachea was deviated to the left and the right side of the chest was hyper-resonant.

87.   A driver of a classic sports car is involved in a head-on impact. On examination he is short of breath and a part of his right hemithorax moves in on inspiration and out on expiration.

88.   A patient who sustained blunt trauma is brought to A&E. She is short of breath, cyanotic and has extensive cervical surgical emphysema.

Theme: Colorectal operations

Options:

a   Pan-proctocolectomy
b   Extended right hemicolectomy
c   Transverse colectomy
d   Subtotal colectomy
e   Extended left hemicolectomy
f   Anterior resection of the rectum
g   Abdominoperineal resection of the rectum

For each of the case scenarios below, choose the single most likely option from the list above. Each option may be used once, more than once or not at all.

89.   A woman in her thirties with fulminant Crohn's colitis which is not responding to medical treatment.

90.   A 63-year-old man with an adenocarcinoma 8 cm from the anal margin.

91.   A 67-year-old woman with a distal transverse colon carcinoma.

Theme: Suture material

Options:

a   2/0 polyamide (nylon)
b   0 polyamide
c   3/0 polypropylene (prolene)
d   2/0 polyglactin (vicryl)
e   4/0 polyglactin
f   6/0 polypropylene
g   3/0 catgut

For each of the case scenarios below, choose the single most likely option from the list above. Each option may be used once, more than once or not at all.

92.   Bowel anastomosis following extended right hemicolectomy.

93.   Anastomosis of the internal thoracic artery to the left anterior descending artery.

94.   Repair of abdominal aortic aneurysm.

95.   Abdominal wall closure.

Theme: Abnormal cardiac pressure measurement

Options:
a   Mitral regurgitation
b   Cardiogenic shock
c   Tricuspid regurgitation
d   Aortic stenosis
e   Aortic regurgitation
f   Dissecting thoracic aneurysm
g   Pulmonary hypertension

For each of the case scenarios below, choose the single most likely option from the list above. Each option may be used once, more than once or not at all.

96. Aortic pressure of 145/45 mmHg.
97. Left ventricular pressure of 180/10 mmHg and aortic pressure of 130/85 mmHg.

Theme: Triage according to need of treatment

Options:
a   X, Y then Z
b   X, Z then Y
c   Y, X then Z
d   Y, Z then X
e   Z, X then Y
f   Z, Y then X

For each of the case scenarios below, choose the single most likely option from the list above. Each option may be used once, more than once or not at all.

98. Three pedestrians are hit by a car: X is unconscious and apnoeic at times; pulse 130 bpm, BP 95/60 mmHg. Y is bleeding profusely from an arm wound; pulse 140 bpm, BP 80/45 mmHg. Z is schizophrenic with skull laceration and GCS of 13; pulse 100 bpm, BP 125/90 mmHg.
99. Blast victims: X is pregnant in active labour; RR 24 per minute, pulse 110 bpm, BP 110/70 mmHg. Y is short of breath and has soot around his mouth and on his face, and there is also reduced air entry on the right side; RR 30 per minute, pulse 130 bpm, BP 110/70 mmHg. Z is screaming in pain; he has an angulated femur and a large thigh wound. His leg appears pale; pulse 140 bpm, BP 85/45 mmHg.
100. Car crash: X is the driver who has a distended abdomen; pulse 120 bpm, BP 90/55 mmHg. He is complaining of severe pain radiating to the left shoulder. Y was thrown out of the car. She is unconscious with a RR 30 per minute, pulse 120 bpm. The right hemithorax is hyper-resonant and the trachea is deviated to the left. Z has severe facial injury and continues to bleed from the mouth and nose. He appears cyanotic; pulse 130 bpm, BP 100/60 mmHg, RR 40 per minute.

Theme: Lung disease

Options:

a   Emphysema
b   Bronchiectasis
c   Asthma
d   Pancoast tumour
e   Fibrosing alveolitis
f   Chronic bronchitis
g   Pulmonary TB

For each of the case scenarios below, choose the single most likely option from the list above. Each option may be used once, more than once or not at all.

101. A 35-year-old woman is admitted for cholecystectomy. She is known to have lung disease and lung function tests revealed (normal range in brackets): FEV_1 2 (3–4), FVC 4 (3.7–5) and PEFR of 150 and 410 after bronchodilator.

102. A 65-year-old woman is admitted for total hip replacement. She is known to have lung disease, therefore a lung function test was performed. This showed: FEV_1 1.5 and FVC 1.9. Her total lung capacity is 40% of normal.

Theme: Nipple discharge

Options:

a   Physiological
b   Mammary duct fistula
c   Cancer
d   Intraductal papilloma
e   Mammary dysplasia
f   Duct ectasia
g   Galactocoele

For each of the case scenarios below, choose the single most likely option from the list above. Each option may be used once, more than once or not at all.

103. A woman in her sixties presents with bloody discharge from the nipple. Attempts at expressing discharge by the examining clinician fail but a mammogram reveals an area of microcalcification.

104. A multiparous woman in her forties presents with clear discharge from the breast. An USS and a mammogram reveal no abnormality.

105. A woman in her early sixties presents with a green nipple discharge. A mammogram shows dilated and calcified ducts.

ANSWERS TO PRACTICE PAPER THREE

The letters of the correct answers are given

MCQs

1.   The following are tumour suppressor genes
A, B, C, D
The K-*ras* gene is an oncogene.

2.   Chest radiograph
B, C, D
The right heart border is formed by the right atrium. The left atrial appendage is usually visible on a PA film.

3.   Pressure measurements in normal heart chambers
B, C, D
The normal right atrial pressure is about 0–4 mmHg. The diastolic pressure in the left ventricle is 0–10 mmHg.

4.   Regarding haemorrhagic shock in an average adult
B, C, D, F
Class I is the loss of up to 15% of circulating blood volume. In class II (15–30%) there is narrowing of the pulse pressure as the diastolic pressure rises and the systolic pressure remains stable.

5.   Regarding haemophilia (A and B)
A, C
Haemophilia A is also known as factor VIII deficiency, whereas haemophilia B is due to factor IX deficiency and called Christmas disease. Both have sex-linked inheritance. They are treated with the relevant clotting factor.

6.   The following variables are used to calculate pH
A, E
According to the formula: $pH = pKa + Log ([HCO_3^-]/[CO_2])$.

7.   The following are Gram-positive rods
B, E

8.   Regarding surgical patients on long-term steroid therapy
All true

9. The following states are associated with compromised immunity
All true
There are many other factors including drugs, haematological disorders, chronic medical disorders such as diabetes and the inflammatory response to surgery and trauma.

10. The following factors increase the risk of wound infection
All true

11. Regarding interosseous needle in children with trauma
E only
An interosseous needle is usually inserted into the tibia or femur if attempts at venous catheterization have failed. Crystalloids, colloids and drugs can be given in this way with a reasonably fast circulation time which is less than 30 seconds.

12. Regarding bowel anastomosis
C, D
A single layer anastomosis involving the seromuscular layer only is recommended.

13. The following are advantages of epidural over spinal anaesthesia
A, B, E
Both types of block affect the sympathetic nerves first due to their small diameter. This results in loss of peripheral vascular tone and precipitous hypotension especially in hypovolaemic patients. Epidural analgesia produces less profound hypotension. Headache occurs in 1–3% of patients after spinal anaesthesia due to CSF leak which is more common than after epidural. Spinal anesthesia is usually a single bolus procedure although a fine catheter can be used for postoperative pain relief.

14. Regarding diathermy
C, E
The electric current passes between the two poles of the forceps in bipolar diathermy and through the patient's body in monopolar diathermy. A plate is used in the case of monopolar diathermy which is required to be at least $70\,cm^2$ in surface area. Diathermy operates at higher frequency ($>400\,kHz$) than domestic mains ($50\,Hz$) and therefore does not affect the neuromuscular junction. This prevents electrocution.

15. Sterilization by steam
C only
Steam is very effective at transferring its latent heat to microorganisms and spores. It therefore sterilizes instruments at a lower temperature and in a shorter time period than dry heat. The steam autoclave is designed to generate supra-atmospheric pressures for water to attain a temperature higher than its boiling point. Dry heat is more suitable for sterilizing non-aqueous liquids.

16. The intracellular compartment in a 70 kg male
A, E
The intracellular and extracellular compartments have the same osmolality at

equilibrium. The chief *anion* here is potassium whereas 95% of sodium is extracellular. Water movement across the cell membrane is regulated by osmotic pressure and active Na/K pump.

17. Blunt trauma to the spleen
A, B, C, D

18. Donated blood is screened for
C, D, E, F
Cytomegalovirus is tested for if blood is to be given to high-risk patients, i.e. immunosuppressed.

19. The following are clinical signs of malnutrition
A, B, D, F
Other signs are gingivitis, glossitis, and prominent bones and tendons.

20. The following parameters are set on a PCA syringe driver
A, C, D
A maximum dose limit is set per 4- and 24-hour periods. The patient does not receive any analgesia during sleep or if they are unable to press the button for any reason. PCA may be difficult for elderly patients or those with poor cognitive function to operate.

21. Platelets
A, C, D, E
The life span of platelets is 9–12 days.

22. Metastatic calcification
A, B, C, E
This form of calcification occurs in cases where serum or tissue calcium levels are abnormally elevated.
Calcium is deposited in normal tissues throughout the body.
Psammoma bodies represent a form of dystrophic calcification which occurs in abnormal tissue.

23. The following disorders are thought to be autoimmune
A, B, C, E
De Quervain's thyroiditis is thought to be viral in origin.

24. Methods of maintaining a patent airway in the traumatized patient
B, C
It is recommended not to pass any tube or catheter nasally if a fracture of the base of the skull is suspected. Oropharyngeal airway in the conscious patient will induce vomiting with risk of subsequent aspiration. An emergency surgical airway is limited to cricothyroidotomy.

25. Flail chest
A, D

The hypoxia occurs because of the extensive lung damage rather than the impaired ventilation. Most cases are treated with pain relief and physiotherapy. Ventilation is indicated if the patient is hypoxic.

26. Methods employed for emergency splintage of a fracture in a patient with multiple trauma
C, D, E

27. The following are recognized complications of burns
All true

Renal failure occurs because of disturbance of fluid balance and hypoperfusion in addition to toxic byproducts of tissue necrosis. Inhalation injury leads to oedema of the larynx and airway resulting in obstruction. Further respiratory embarrassment may result in the presence of circumferential thoracic burns.

28. Cardiac action potential
A, B, C

Slow-response fibres have a longer relative refractory period which extends into phase 4, i.e. after full repolarization of the fibre.

The steep upstroke of the fast response is due to the influx of Na^+ through the fast Na^+ channels.

29. Surface markings of diaphragmatic openings
A only

The aortic hiatus is about 2.5 cm above the transpyloric plane in the midline. The oesophageal hiatus is at the level of the 7th costal cartilage but lies about 2.5 cm to the left of the midline.

30. Carcinoma of the bronchus may present with
A, B, D, E

Oat cell tumours may present with Cushing's syndrome not disease.

31. The following layers are encountered on inserting a subclavian venous line
A, B, D

The layers in order are skin, fat or superficial fascia, deep fascia, pectoralis major, clavipectoral fascia and subclavius.

32. Indications for dialysis include
B, D, E

Other indications are hyperkalaemia not responding to other measures and encephalopathy.

33. The following are used to calculate the APACHE score
A, C, D, E

Others include: pulse, BP, RR, pH, PaO_2, haematocrit, potassium, creatinine, age, emergency vs. elective operation and other chronic diseases.

34. The following nerves traverse the diaphragm
A, D, E
The lesser and least splanchnic nerves also traverse the diaphragm by piercing the crura on either side.

35. The following constitute paraneoplastic syndromes
A, B
This is a group of symptoms that can not be readily explained by local or distant spread of tumour or the production of hormones indigenous to the tissue from which the tumour originated.

36. Factors that contribute to development of the adult female breast at puberty
B, C, D, E, F

37. Brain abscess
C, E
Brain abscesses occur mostly in patients with sepsis elsewhere, usually the chest, abdomen, sinuses and ears. The temporal and frontal lobes are most commonly affected. They present with deterioration of conscious level, focal signs and epilepsy. A short history of presentation is associated with generalized inflammation and worse oedema, and these patients tend to do badly.

38. The following are recognized eye signs in hyperthyroidism
A, D, E
Other signs are lid retraction and exophthalmos.

39. Hernias around the umbilicus
A, C
Umbilical hernias in children do not require surgery unless they present with obstruction or strangulation. Adult paraumbilical hernias should be repaired surgically because of the ever present risk of strangulation as they tend to have a narrow neck.

40. The following examinations are necessary before urethral catheterization of a trauma patient
A, B, E
Integrity of the urethra must be sought before passing a catheter.

41. The following are recognized methods of treating chronic pancreatitis
A, B, C, E
A patient with chronic pancreatitis should be managed conservatively by a multidisciplinary team. Surgery is reserved for those with intractable pain or the development of complications requiring surgery.

42. Blind loop syndrome
A, B

This is due to bacterial overgrowth in a defunctioned part of the bowel which results in malabsorption. The patient usually presents with diarrhoea and weight loss. Steatorrhoea may also be present and there may be vitamin B_{12} deficiency and anaemia.

43. BRCA1 gene
B, C, E

44. The following organisms cause opportunistic infections
All true

The group above encompasses bacteria, fungi and parasites. Viruses such as cytomegalovirus, herpes simplex and herpes zoster can also cause opportunistic infections.

45. Recognized complications of insertion of a central venous catheter include
A, C, E

Other complications include haemorrhage, haematoma, pneumothorax and injury to other neck and mediastinal structures. Late complications include infection and thromboembolism.

46. Transfusion with fresh frozen plasma is indicated to correct
C, D, E

An elevated INR in the absence of haemorrhage can be corrected with vitamin K administration unless emergency surgery is anticipated.

47. Traumatic diaphragmatic rupture
C only

Diaphragmatic rupture is commonest on the left side and is rarely bilateral. The diagnosis is easy to miss but the presence of a gastric bubble and an elevated right hemidiaphragm on CXR are two of the common signs.

48. Base of skull fractures
A, B, C, D

49. Values measured on spirometry
A, E

Measuring the FEV_1/FVC is useful in differentiating restrictive from obstructive ventilatory defects.

50. The following are useful prognostic factors in breast cancer
All true

EMQs

Theme: Definition of statistical terms used in medicine
61-e Also known as the validity of the test.
62-b
63-d Attributable risk is rate of disease in the exposed — rate of disease in the unexposed.

Theme: Treatment of obstructive jaundice
64-d This patient's disease cannot be resected for cure. The jaundice can be effectively palliated with a stent.
65-a This patient is suitable for a Whipple's procedure if he is medically fit.
66-e Another strategy of managing these patients is laparoscopic cholecystectomy with exploration of the common bile duct.

Theme: Immediate management of thoracic trauma
67-b There is a high risk of right ventricular injury. This patient may have a tamponade that needs to be relieved immediately before emergency thoracotomy to repair any cardiac injury preferably with the provision of cardiopulmonary bypass.
68-a This woman is likely to have haemothorax.
69-g Blood transfusion and observation is all that is needed at this stage. Continuing loss of > 200 ml/hour makes a thoracotomy mandatory.

Theme: Sterilization and disinfection of surgical instruments
70-c This is effective and fast. Non-stainless metal and delicate instruments can be sterilized in a dry heat autoclave which takes a longer time and employs higher temperatures.
71-f Other latex material such as urinary catheters and i.v. giving sets are sterilized in this way.
72-e Immersion in glutaraldehyde or boiling water is a method of disinfection rather than sterilization.
73-d

Theme: The person capable of giving informed consent
74-c Although adolescents have the right to accept surgery, those under 18 cannot refuse life-saving surgery and the parents can consent to the procedure.
75-a Even those under section to receive psychiatric treatment cannot be forced to have surgical procedures for physical conditions.
76-d Although the attending doctor can not act as the patient's proxy, in this case they have a legal and moral duty to treat the patient rendering consent unnecessary.

Theme: Nutritional support
77-e This kind of tube is inserted beyond the anastomosis at the time of surgery and can be used to feed patients early.

78-b Until the fistula heals if being treated conservatively.

79-c Established endoscopically, this a good route for providing long-term nutrition.

Theme: Pain relief

80-f Good pain control in patients with abdominal and thoracic incisions prevents the development of serious respiratory complications.

81-b Most of these patients are treated as day cases. Local anaesthetic injection into the wound and this analgesic regime are usually adequate. Weak opiates may be added to this combination.

82-e A continuous opiate infusion can also be used.

Theme: Structures injured during surgery on the neck

83-c This is a manifestation of hypocalcaemia.

84-b Injury to this nerve, which supplies the cricothyroid muscle, produces a subtle deficit.

85-e This is Horner's syndrome.

Theme: Thoracic trauma

86-d

87-a These patients suffer from hypoventilation due to paradoxical movement and pulmonary contusion which has more of an adverse effect on their respiration than hypoventilation. Pain relief may improve the patient's ventilation but some will need mechanical ventilation.

88-c Damage to the airways proximal to the pleural reflection presents with surgical emphysema whereas damage distal to the pleural reflection presents with pneumothorax. Bronchoscopy to assess the damage followed by surgical repair are indicated in this patient.

Theme: Colorectal operations

89-d An end ileostomy is formed at the time of surgery, with a possibility of reversal if restorative proctectomy is performed at a later stage.

90-f A tumour at this distance allows the minimum distal margin of 2 cm and preservation of the anal sphincter mechanism.

91-e The standard left hemicolectomy does not extend beyond the splenic flexure proximally.

Theme: Suture material

92-d 3/0 PDS may also be used.

93-f

94-c

95-b

Theme: Abnormal cardiac pressure measurement

96-e This patient has severe aortic regurgitation. The pulse pressure of 100 mmHg is an indication for surgery.

97-a A gradient of more than 50 mmHg is an indication for surgery.

Theme: Triage according to need of treatment

98-a Triage of a group of patients is similar to treating a single patient, i.e. serious injury is treated first following the **A**irway, **B**reathing and **C**irculation dogma. X has an **A**irway problem. Y has a **C**irculatory problem. Z has a neurological **D**ysfunction problem.

99-d Y has an **A**irway and a **B**reathing problem. Z has a **C**irculatory problem. X's problem is not immediately life threatening.

100-f Z has Airway and Circulatory problems at least. Y has a **B**reathing problem. X has a **C**irculatory problem.

Theme: Lung disease

101-c This is a picture of obstructive airway disease. The $FEV_1/FVC < 75\%$, and the low PEFR is reversed with bronchodilators.

102-e This woman has restrictive lung disease as the $FEV_1/FEV \geqslant 75\%$. She is likely to have impaired CO gas transfer.

Theme: Nipple discharge

103-c Another cause of bloody discharge is intraductal papilloma.

104-a

105-f Green discharge also occurs around the menopause.

PRACTICE PAPER ONE: SYSTEM MODULES

MCQs

1. Haemorrhoids

A   Are termed second degree when they prolapse permanently
B   Often present with pruritus ani
C   Are termed proctalgia fugax when painful
D   Are best treated with haemorrhoidectomy if third degree

2. Benign prostatic hypertrophy

A   Increases in incidence with age
B   Is associated with a hard texture and obliteration of the median sulcus on palpating the prostate through the rectal wall
C   The patient's symptoms correlate with the size of the prostate
D   5-α-Reductase inhibitors relieve symptoms by relaxing the bladder neck
E   May be complicated by retrograde ejaculation

3. Carcinoma of the stomach

A   Occurs most commonly in the fundus
B   Signet ring cells, when present, indicate a poor prognosis
C   Is more common in patients with pernicious anaemia
D   Has decreased in incidence in the UK and USA over the last few decades
E   The prognosis depends mostly on the grade of the malignancy and not the stage of the disease

4. Femoral hernia

A   Is usually lateral to the femoral vein
B   Can be repaired be suturing the inguinal ligament to the lacunar ligament
C   Can be left untreated in the elderly thin female
D   Can be difficult to distinguish from an inguinal hernia

5. **Conditions presenting with bilious vomiting include**

A Intussusception
B Duodenal atresia
C Meconium ileus
D Oesophageal atresia
E Midgut volvulus

6. **Carcinoma of the oral cavity**

A Is predominantly adenocarcinoma in type
B Is associated with smoking
C Can metastasize to bilateral cervical lymph nodes
D Is associated with excessive exposure to sunlight
E The size of the tumour and the stage determine the prognosis

7. **The following are risk factors for atherosclerosis**

A Diabetes mellitus
B Older age
C Age at menarche
D Hyperuricaemia
E Strong family history
F Radiotherapy for breast cancer
G Body mass index

8. **The foramen of Winslow**

A Is the only communication between the lesser sac and the peritoneal cavity
B Has the pylorus as its inferior border
C Has the caudate process of the liver as its superior border
D Is limited anteriorly by the free edge of the lesser omentum
E Is bounded by two veins; the portal vein anteriorly and the inferior vena cava posteriorly

9. **The following are recognized complications of Colles' fracture**

A Extensor digiti minimi rupture
B Malunion
C Extensor pollicis longus tendon rupture

D   Reflex sympathetic dystrophy
E   Radial head subluxation
F   Carpal tunnel syndrome

10.   Regarding the order in which layers are incised when approaching the thyroid gland

A   Skin, platysma, pretracheal fascia and strap muscles
B   Skin, platysma, deep cervical fascia, areolar tissue between the strap muscles followed by pretracheal fascia
C   Skin, deep cervical fascia, platysma, areolar tissue between the strap muscles followed by strap muscles and pretracheal fascia
D   Skin, platysma, deep cervical fascia, areolar tissue between the strap muscles and prevertebral fascia
E   Skin, platysma, pretracheal fascia, strap muscles and deep cervical fascia

11.   With regard to vascular imaging

A   Intra-arterial digital subtraction angiography (IA DSA) is the preferred method for imaging below the knee
B   Intravenous DSA is safer than IA DSA in patients with borderline renal function
C   IV DSA is used in patients who will need a therapeutic intervention at the time of the angiography
D   Duplex scanning is the best modality to investigate the iliac arteries
E   Duplex scanning is a combination of B-mode and Doppler ultrasound
F   A good left ventricular ejection fraction is necessary to obtain good images with IV DSA

12.   The following are recognized complications of TB of the spine

A   Bony destruction and paraplegia
B   Kyphosis
C   Malignant transformation
D   Lumbar abscess formation

13.   The adductor canal

A   Starts at the apex of the femoral triangle
B   The roof is formed by gracilis
C   Contains the femoral artery, vein and nerve
D   The floor is formed by adductor longus and magnus
E   Terminates at the hiatus in adductor magnus

14. Congenital dislocation of the hip

A   Occurs more commonly in girls
B   Can be diagnosed clinically using Tinel's test
C   Is usually diagnosed on USS
D   Is associated with breech delivery
E   Does not have a familial tendency

15. Regarding the urethra

A   It consists of two parts
B   The prostatic part is the widest
C   It receives most of its blood supply from the urethral artery
D   It is easiest to dilate in its membranous part
E   There is a 90° angle between the prostatic and membranous urethra

16. The following features are more common in ulcerative colitis than Crohn's disease

A   Pain
B   Transmural inflammation
C   Skip lesions
D   Weight loss and malnutrition
E   Ileal involvement

17. The abdominal aorta

A   Enters the abdomen at the level of T1
B   Is encircled by the two diaphragmatic crura as it enters the abdomen
C   Bifurcates at a point just below the umbilicus and to the left of the midline
D   The origin of the superior mesenteric artery lies posterior to the 3rd part of the duodenum
E   Has five paired lumbar branches supplying the five lumbar vertebrae
F   The celiac trunk is its 1st visceral branch
G   Lies to the left and anterior to the inferior vena cava at the level of L4

18. The knee joint

A   Is a typical synovial joint of the hinge variety
B   The posterior capsule is strengthened by the oblique popliteal ligament laterally
C   The menisci are crescent-shaped structures made of hyaline cartilage
D   The tibial nerve lies against the posterior capsule
E   The anterior cruciate ligament is attached to the posterior and medial surface of the lateral femoral condyle

19. **The following are recognized complications of varicose veins**

A   Rupture and bleeding of varicosities
B   Fistula formation
C   Superficial thrombophlebitis
D   Skin pigmentation
E   Cerebrovascular accidents
F   Skin ulceration

20. **Epiglottitis**

A   Presents with stridor and drooling
B   Occurs most commonly in the age group 15–18
C   The causative organism is *Staphylococcus aureus*
D   Is easily diagnosed by the inexperienced with indirect laryngoscopy
E   The condition responds to amoxycillin

21. **The systemic vascular resistance (SVR)**

A   Is mostly dependent on the diameter of the arterioles
B   Is greater if individual resistors are arranged in series rather than parallel
C   Changes in venous capacitance maintain a constant blood pressure during exercise
D   Is equal to the pulmonary vascular resistance
E   Is equal to blood pressure divided by cardiac output

22. **Tennis elbow**

A   Pain is over the origin of wrist flexors
B   Pain can be produced by flexing the wrist while the elbow is extended
C   In most cases the condition resolves with rest and analgesia
D   There is usually a swelling over the lateral epicondyle
E   Operative treatment involves excision of the lateral epicondyle

23. **The subclavian artery**

A   Supplies the brain
B   Has the internal thoracic artery as a branch
C   Supplies the thyroid gland through the superior thyroid artery
D   The right recurrent laryngeal nerve hooks around the right subclavian artery on its way to the larynx
E   The right subclavian is a branch of the arch of the aorta

24. Epistaxis

A May be caused be telangiectasia
B In the young patient is more likely to be venous
C In the elderly the bleed is from Little's area
D Is associated with hypertension
E Cocaine causes vasoconstriction and can stop the bleeding

25. The factors which determine when an arterial stenosis becomes critical include

A The cross-sectional area of the stenosis
B The radius of the stenosis
C The amount of blood flow in the vessel
D Exercise
E The peripheral vascular resistance beyond the stenosis

26. Regarding calcium metabolism

A Vitamin D increases calcium absorption from the intestine
B Calcitonin activates calcium resorption from bone
C Vitamin D is converted from 25-hydroxycholecalciferol to 1,25-dihydroxycholecalciferol in the kidneys
D Parathyroid hormone will correct a state of hypercalcaemia back to normal
E Elevated serum calcium stimulates the production of calcitonin

27. Fluid management in the neonate

A The neonate conserves sodium more avidly than do adults
B The neonate can only concentrate urine to half that of the adult's ability
C The neonate's heart is less able to adjust to changes in vascular volume than the adult's heart
D Absorption via the gastrointestinal tract is equal to that of the adult
E Neonates require more water (per body weight in 24 hours) than adults

28. The anatomical snuff box

A Is bounded by extensor pollicis longus tendon on the ulnar side
B The tendons of extensor pollicis brevis and abductor pollicis longus form the radial border
C The scaphoid and trapezoid bones form most of the floor
D The basilic vein starts here
E Contains the cutaneous branch of the median nerve

29. Popliteal artery aneurysms

A   The popliteal artery is the commonest site for a peripheral aneurysm
B   Are bilateral in 95% of cases
C   The vast majority of cases present with a palpable lump
D   Mostly occur secondary to trauma

30. Carpal tunnel syndrome

A   Can occur secondary to rheumatoid arthritis
B   Produces paraesthesia of the little and ring fingers
C   Should be differentiated from cervical spondylosis of C6 and C7
D   Should be treated surgically in all patients
E   Occurs in both sexes with the same frequency

31. Jaundice in infants can be caused by

A   Biliary atresia
B   Hirschsprung's disease
C   Cytomegalovirus infection
D   Breast milk jaundice
E   Choledochal cyst

32. The spermatic cord contains

A   The testicular artery
B   The ilioinguinal nerve
C   The genital branch of the genitofemoral nerve
D   The ductus deferens
E   The pampiniform plexus
F   The processus vaginalis
G   The inferior epigastric artery

33. Achalasia of the cardia

A   Commonly presents in the elderly
B   Can be mimicked by carcinoma on the cardia
C   Is associated with increased incidence of adenocarcinoma of the oesophagus
D   Can be treated with a Nissen fundoplication
E   Can be associated with lung abscesses

34. The following are complications of Billroth II gastrectomy

A   Postcibal syndrome or dumping
B   Excessive fat absorption and subsequent weight gain
C   Bilious vomiting
D   Steatorrhoea
E   Blind loop syndrome

35. Meckel's diverticulum

A   Is a patent remnant of the urachus
B   Occurs in about 2% of the population
C   May present with rectal bleeding
D   May contain ectopic gastric mucosa
E   Carcinoid tumours are a common complication

36. Renal cell carcinoma

A   Can present with pyrexia of unknown origin
B   May be associated with polycythaemia
C   Can spread to the inferior vena cava
D   Can spread to the gonads
E   Nephrectomy is the treatment of choice regardless of the stage of the disease
F   Chemotherapy can be used to treat symptomatic bone metastases

37. Osteoarthritis (OA)

A   Is divided into primary, secondary and tertiary according to the aetiology
B   X-rays reveal loss of joint space
C   There is periarticular osteoporosis on X-ray
D   Like rheumatoid arthritis the disease also affects the hands
E   Tibial realignment osteotomy can be used to treat a patient with osteoarthritis affecting both tibiofemoral compartments of the knee joint

38. The oesophagus

A   Enters the abdomen through a diaphragmatic orifice at the level of the T8 vertebra
B   Is narrowest about 15 cm from the incisor teeth, at the level of the cricopharyngeal sphincter

C   Has an outermost layer called the serosa

D   Is supplied by the inferior thyroid artery in its upper third

E   Is more closely related to the posterior vagal than anterior vagal nerve in its abdominal course

39.   Arterial wall structure

A   The aorta has a high elastin content

B   The high smooth muscle content of the aorta facilitates continuous blood flow in diastole

C   Medium-sized peripheral vessels contain more collagen than the aorta

D   The elastin:collagen ratio alters with age

40.   The submandibular salivary gland

A   Drains through a duct that leaves the deep part of the gland

B   Is a mixed gland

C   The hypoglossal nerve hooks underneath the duct and then passes medial to it ascending towards the tongue

D   The deep part is sandwiched between the mylohyoid and hyoglossus

E   Is more frequently affected by calculi than the parotid gland

41.   The following substrates are virtually completely reabsorbed from the proximal tubule of the kidney

A   Glucose

B   Sodium

C   Potassium

D   Chloride

E   Amino acids

42.   Primary malignancies associated with secondary deposits in the adrenal gland include

A   Breast

B   Gastric

C   Melanoma

D   Bronchial

E   Colonic

F   Renal

43. Renal anatomy

A   The hilum of the right kidney is higher than that of the left
B   The ureter is the most posterior structure in the hilum
C   The kidneys are enclosed in two layers of fascia
D   The left renal vein runs posterior to the aorta before entering the inferior vena cava
E   The left renal vein receives blood from the left suprarenal gland

44. Acute renal infection

A   Pyonephrosis is best treated with parenteral antibiotics
B   A carbuncle is usually caused by *Staphylococcus aureus* infection
C   A perinephric abscess may rupture into the pleural cavity
D   Most infections ascend from the lower urinary tract
E   Never requires surgical drainage

45. Hydrocele

A   A primary hydrocele is caused by benign conditions such as trauma
B   The fluid collects between the testis and tunica albuginea
C   A secondary hydrocele is treated by Lord's procedure
D   In a young man is unlikely to be idiopathic

46. The following are radiological features of Colles' fracture

A   Distraction
B   Dorsal shift
C   Volar tilt
D   Dorsal tilt
E   Ulnar shift

47. Carotid artery stenosis

A   Accounts for 90% of strokes
B   Carries a 20–30% annual risk of stroke in symptomatic patients with 70% stenosis
C   Is usually investigated with selective carotid angiography
D   Is often treated operatively in asymptomatic patients undergoing cardiac bypass surgery
E   When treated operatively carries a 10% risk of stroke

48. Osteomalacia

A   Results from reduced calcification of osteoid
B   Is usually due to reduced calcium intake
C   Most patients will have hypocalcaemia
D   May be secondary to chronic renal failure

49. Conn's syndrome

A   Is caused by an adrenal adenoma
B   Presents with profound hypotension
C   Frequently presents with hypokalaemia
D   The primary abnormality is hyperaldosteronism
E   Can be treated surgically

50. The following are recognized complications of laparoscopic surgery

A   Increased inflammatory response to surgery
B   Arterial injury
C   Hypocapnia
D   Port site herniation
E   Port site recurrence in cancer surgery

EMQs

Theme: Shoulder conditions

Options:
a   Frozen shoulder
b   Anterior dislocation
c   Posterior dislocation
d   Rotator cuff tear
e   Chronic tendinitis
f   Rheumatoid arthritis
g   Septic arthritis

For each of the case scenarios below, choose the single most likely option from the list above. Each option may be used once, more than once or not at all.

61.   A 22-year-old male presents with a painful left shoulder after an epileptic fit. On examination the arm is held in fixed medial rotation.

62. A 60-year-old porter complains of shoulder pain. It started when lifting a heavy weight 6 months previously. On examination he finds it difficult to abduct his shoulder.

63. A 45-year-old male presents with chronic shoulder pain. He finds it difficult to abduct the arm between 60° and 120°. Abduction in external rotation is much better tolerated.

Theme: Chronic limb ischaemia

Options:
a   Embolectomy
b   Vascular reconstruction
c   Angioplasty
d   Surgical sympathectomy
e   Thrombolysis
f   Prostaglandin infusion
g   Amputation
h   Conservative treatment

For each of the case scenarios below, choose the single most likely option from the list above. Each option may be used once, more than once or not at all.

64. An 80-year-old woman with a 10-year history of claudication presents with severe leg pain which has kept her up at night for the last month. She had a stroke 6 months previously which rendered her immobile and heavily dependent on nursing home staff. Advanced gangrene is evident.

65. A 50-year-old smoker presents with claudication pain of 4 months duration. The pain comes after walking about 400 yards uphill. There is no history of diabetes and his father died of myocardial infarction.

66. A 60-year-old ex-smoker presents with rest pain. His claudication has been getting worse over the last 6 months. Investigations show a 9 cm long occluded femoropopliteal segment.

Theme: Conditions that cause splenomegaly

Options:
a   Portal hypertension
b   Glandular fever
c   Bacterial endocarditis
d   Chronic myeloid leukaemia
e   Hodgkin's disease
f   Malaria
g   Sarcoid

For each of the case scenarios below, choose the single most likely option from the list above. Each option may be used once, more than once or not at all.

67. Solomon is a 10-year-old boy. He has been unwell for 1 week. His main complaints are intermittent fever and headache. Six weeks ago he returned from Nigeria where he visited his grandmother. On examination his temperature is 40°C and he has mild splenomegaly.

68. A 40-year-old man presents with abdominal pain. His health has deteriorated over the past 4 months with significant weight loss and recurrent fever. On examination his spleen and liver are enlarged and his spleen is tender on palpation. There is no lymphadenopathy.

69. A 60-year-old homeless man is brought into A&E having been found unconscious. There is altered blood on his clothes and in his mouth. He smells of alcohol and is jaundiced with a distended abdomen and an enlarged spleen.

Theme: Ear and throat conditions

Options:
a   Tonsillitis
b   Acute mastoiditis
c   Otitis externa
d   Herpes zoster
e   Furunculosis
f   Acute otitis media
g   Traumatic tympanic membrane perforation

For each of the case scenarios below, choose the single most likely option from the list above. Each option may be used once, more than once or not at all.

70. A 7-year-old boy presents with severe left ear pain. His temperature is 38.5°C, the pinna is not inflamed and there is no discharge.

71. A 13-year-old girl with a 1-week history of ear pain and purulent discharge presents with deteriorating hearing deficit and headache. On examination the pinna is displaced forwards and downwards and there is significant postauricular tenderness.

72. A 4-year-old girl presents with a 2-day history of bilateral ear pain, fever and painful swallowing.

Theme: Cervical lymphadenopathy

Options:
a   Submandibular
b   Jugulodigastric

c   Upper deep cervical
d   Middle deep cervical
e   Left supraclavicular
f   Occipital
g   Submental
h   Preauricular

For each of the case scenarios below, choose the single most likely option from the list above. Each option may be used once, more than once or not at all.

73.   Mr B. Lee is 56. He is a businessman from Hong Kong on holiday in the UK. He presents with a 4-month history of blood-stained discharge from his right nostril and deafness of the right ear.

74.   Mr Davies is a 67-year-old retired miner. He complains of an ulcer on the tip of his tongue which has not improved over the past 4 months. His fingers are heavily stained by tobacco.

75.   Simon is 19 years old. He noticed that his right testis was enlarged when he sustained a minor injury while playing football. An ultrasound scan confirms that the appearance is compatible with malignancy.

76.   A 70-year-old ex-builder presents with squamous cell carcinoma of the scalp 3 cm behind his ear.

Theme: Aortoiliac atherosclerosis

Options:
a   Angioplasty
b   Extravascular stenting
c   Aortobifemoral bypass
d   Axillobifemoral bypass
e   Femoropopliteal bypass
f   Endarterectomy
g   Amputation

For each of the case scenarios below, choose the single most likely option from the list above. Each option may be used once, more than once or not at all.

77.   A 75-year-old man presents with severe, bilateral aortoiliac occlusion. The atheromatous lesion is rather diffuse. He has severe emphysema and a history of two myocardial infarctions. He has developed rest pain in both lower limbs.

78.   A 60-year-old smoker presents with severe stenosis of his right common iliac artery. The stenotic lesion is 4 cm long and the patient has been unable to work for 6 months due to leg pain.

79.   A 63-year-old man presents with a lesion similar to that of the 75-year-old patient above. He has no significant medical history and he stopped smoking 5 years ago. He is now unable to play golf or walk long distances.

Theme: Hoarse voice

Options:

a   Laryngitis
b   Swallowed foreign body
c   External laryngeal nerve palsy
d   Laryngeal cancer
e   Thyroid cancer
f   TB
g   Carcinoma of the bronchus

For each of the case scenarios below, choose the single most likely option from the list above. Each option may be used once, more than once or not at all.

80.   A 63-year-old smoker with a long history of peptic ulcer disease and ischaemic heart disease presents with 1 month's history of hoarse voice that has been getting progressively worse.

81.   A 65-year-old woman presents with hoarse voice. She has been unwell for the last 3 months and lost 7 kg in weight. She also complains of persistent cough productive of a small amount of blood. She has smoked 15 cigarettes a day for 45 years.

Theme: Bone 'tumours'

Options:

a   Chondroma
b   Ewing's sarcoma
c   Osteochondroma
d   Bone cyst
e   Osteosarcoma
f   Osteoid osteoma
g   Multiple myeloma

For each of the case scenarios below, choose the single most likely option from the list above. Each option may be used once, more than once or not at all.

82.   A 10-year-old girl falls and fractures her left femur. X-ray examination reveals a well-demarcated lucent area through which the proximal femur fractured.

83.   A 15-year-old boy presents with a painful right femoral lesion. On examination the lump is ill defined, hot and tender. Radiographs of the area in question show bony destruction and overlying periosteal new bone giving an onion skin appearance.

84.   A 75-year-old woman with Paget's disease develops a painful lump in her right tibia. The pain is different to that caused by Paget's disease. On examination there is a tender and ill-defined lump.

Theme: Causes of right iliac fossa pain

Options:
a   Mesenteric adenitis
b   Ruptured ectopic pregnancy
c   Appendicitis
d   Ureteric colic
e   Torsion of ovarian cyst
f   Pelvic inflammatory disease
g   Inflamed Meckel's diverticulum
h   Crohn's disease

For each of the case scenarios below, choose the single most likely option from the list above. Each option may be used once, more than once or not at all.

85.   A 7-year-old girl presents with a 1-day history of pain associated with anorexia and one episode of diarrhoea.
86.   A 25-year-old male presents with a 6-month history of weight loss. There is a mass in the right iliac fossa.
87.   A 21-year-old female presents with acute onset of severe pain and feeling clammy and unwell. On examination there is marked tenderness. The pregnancy test is negative.

Theme: Abdominal distension

Options:
a   Small bowel obstruction
b   Large bowel obstruction
c   Perforated duodenal ulcer
d   Acute intestinal ischaemia
e   Pseudo-obstruction
f   Sigmoid volvulus
g   Ascites

For each of the case scenarios below, choose the single most likely option from the list above. Each option may be used once, more than once or not at all

88.   A male prison inmate, aged 36, is brought to A&E. He was found collapsed in his cell. On examination he is comatose and hypotensive. The abdomen is very distended and tympanitic. There is no dullness to percussion over the liver and the bowel sounds are absent.
89.   A 75-year-old patient with Parkinson's disease presents with progressive abdominal distension over a period of 3 months. He has not opened his bowels for 1 week. On examination he has a tympanitic abdomen which is non-tender and normal bowel sounds. An abdominal film reveals gas in the rectum.

90. The duty psychiatrist refers a woman, aged 81, with dementia. She presents with acutely developed abdominal pain, distension, vomiting and absolute constipation. The abdominal radiograph reveals a distended Ω-shaped large bowel loop arising from the pelvis.

Theme: Carcinoma of the bladder

Options:

a   Cystectomy
b   External beam radiotherapy
c   Intravesical chemotherapy
d   Pelvic lymphadenectomy
e   Transurethral resection of tumour
f   Systemic chemotherapy
g   Orchidectomy

For each of the case scenarios below, choose the single most likely option from the list above. Each option may be used once, more than once or not at all.

91. A 62-year-old factory worker presents with haematuria. Investigation reveals a tumour which is believed to be confined to the mucosa.
92. A 79-year-old man presents with haematuria. He has a history of ischaemic heart disease and chronic obstructive pulmonary disease. The histology of the resected bladder tumour found on cystoscopy shows invasive carcinoma.
93. A 47-year-old man presents with frequency and urgency. There is microscopic haematuria but all microbiological cultures have been negative. On cystoscopy the whole of the bladder mucosa was inflamed and the bladder volume was reduced.

Theme: Vomiting

Options:

a   Strangulated hernia
b   Gastric volvulus
c   Adhesive obstruction
d   Pyloric stenosis
e   Achalasia
f   Caecal carcinoma
g   Gastroenteritis

For each of the case scenarios below, choose the single most likely option from the list above. Each option may be used once, more than once or not at all.

94. A 35-year-old woman presents with vomiting and increasing tenderness around the umbilicus. She underwent a negative gynaecological laparoscopy 4 days earlier.

95. A 55-year-old man presents with profuse vomiting over 2 days. He is a known epileptic and has suffered with duodenal ulcer in the past. On examination he has no abdominal distension or signs of peritonitis. His serum chemistry shows hypokalaemia and his pH is 7.52.

Theme: Treatment of conditions of the thyroid

Options:

a   Radioactive iodine
b   Thyroxine replacement
c   Subtotal thyroidectomy
d   Total thyroidectomy, lymph node clearance, thyroxine replacement and radioactive iodine
e   Iodine supplement
f   Thyroid lobectomy
g   Total thyroidectomy and thyroxine replacement

For each of the case scenarios below, choose the single most likely option from the list above. Each option may be used once, more than once or not at all.

96. A 23-year-old female presents with a lump in her thyroid. The lump is 'cold' on the isotope scan and an ultrasound scan shows it to be 3 cm in diameter. FNA confirms the presence of papillary carcinoma. At the time of surgery there is evidence of lymph node involvement and the frozen section shows a papillary carcinoma that has invaded the thyroid capsule.

97. A 31-year-old lawyer with Grave's disease had a 6-month course of carbimazole. Unfortunately, her symptoms recurred within 3 months of cessation of treatment. She plans to get married and start a family in 1 year's time.

98. Five years post subtotal thyroidectomy for a benign thyroid condition a patient presents with depression, weight gain and lethargy. Her TSH is elevated.

Theme: Scrotal conditions in adults

Options:

a   Epididymal cyst
b   Inguinoscrotal hernia
c   Torsion of the testis
d   Testicular tumour
e   Varicocele
f   Hydrocele
g   Orchitis

For each of the case scenarios below, choose the single most likely option from the list above. Each option may be used once, more than once or not at all.

99. A 63-year-old man with right-sided testicular swelling. This has been present for 18 months. On examination it is not possible 'to get above' the swelling.

100. A 29-year-old man presents with a 1-week history of heavy and tender left testis. On examination the right testis is normal in size but harder and slightly more tender to palpate than the left testis. The cord and epididymis are normal.

101. A 36-year-old man presents with a dragging sensation and swelling in the scrotum. On examination the testes are normal but he has what feels like 'a bag of worms' on the left side.

102. An elderly man presents with change in bowel habit. Routine examination of the scrotum reveals a 2 cm swelling above and behind the testis. The testis feels normal.

Theme: Fractured neck of femur

Options:
a   Skeletal traction
b   Hemiarthroplasty
c   Dynamic hip screw
d   Cast brace
e   Bipolar hemiarthroplasty
f   External fixation
g   Skin traction

For each of the case scenarios below, choose the single most likely option from the list above. Each option may be used once, more than once or not at all.

103. An 85-year-old woman, previously mobile without aid, fell while gardening and sustained a Garden grade 3 transcervical fracture of the neck of her right femur.

104. A 63-year-old fit woman sustained a Garden grade 4 subcapital fracture.

105. A 75-year-old woman presents with an intertrochanteric fracture.

ANSWERS TO PRACTICE PAPER ONE

The letters of the correct answers are given

MCQs

1. Haemorrhoids
B, D

Third-degree haemorrhoids remain prolapsed permanently. Pain is not a feature of uncomplicated piles and the term proctalgia fugax is used to describe a condition of severe anal pain of unclear aetiology.

2. Benign prostatic hypertrophy
A only

The patient's complaint is not related to the size of the prostate. On examination the prostate feels firm with a palpable median sulcus. Medical treatment includes 5-α-reductase inhibitors which reduce the gland size by interfering with testosterone metabolism. α-Adrenergic blocking agents work by relaxing the bladder neck. The mainstay of surgical treatment is TURP. This can be complicated by retrograde ejaculation.

3. Carcinoma of the stomach
B, C, D

Carcinoma of the stomach occurs most commonly in the gastric antrum and body. The prognosis is closely linked to the stage of the disease where early tumours, i.e. not invading the muscularis propria, carry the best prognosis.

4. Femoral hernia
D

A femoral hernia is usually medial to the femoral vein. Expeditious repair should be undertaken in all cases because of the high incidence of strangulation and the morbidity associated with an emergency operation. This can be done by suturing the inguinal ligament to the pectineal ligament.

5. Conditions presenting with bilious vomiting include
A, B, C, E

Obstruction proximal to the second part of the duodenum produces vomiting which is not bile-stained.

6. Carcinoma of the oral cavity
B, C, D, E

The vast majority of oral malignancies are squamous cell carcinoma in type. These are associated with smoking (especially pipe smoking), human papilloma virus infection, prolonged exposure to sunlight (in lip cancer) and heavy alcoholic intake. Tumours in the midline and posterior aspect of the tongue metastasize to nodes in both sides of the neck.

7. The following are risk factors for atherosclerosis
All true except C

8. The foramen of Winslow
A, C, D, E
The inferior border of the foramen of Winslow is formed by the 1st part of the duodenum.

9. The following are recognized complications of Colles' fracture
B, C, D, F
Other complications include radioulnar joint subluxation and stiffness.

10. Regarding the order in which layers are incised when approaching the thyroid gland
B

11. With regard to vascular imaging
A, E, F
Duplex scanning is an inexpensive and non-invasive way of investigating vascular disorders. However, images can be of poor quality if the vessels are obscured by bowel gas. IV DSA is a less invasive method of angiography than IA DSA, but images are poor both in the presence of heart failure and if the vessels investigated are distal. The large dose of contrast needed makes it contraindicated in borderline renal function. IA DSA can be used for diagnosis and treatment at the same time.

12. The following are recognized complications of TB of the spine
A, B, D

13. The adductor canal
A, D, E
This is also known as the subsartorial canal due to the fact that the sartorius forms its roof. The contents of the canal are the femoral vessels and the saphenous nerve. The nerve to vastus medialis travels a short course in the canal.

14. Congenital dislocation of the hip
A, C, D
This condition occurs eight times more commonly in girls. Both genetic and environmental factors are implicated in its pathogenesis. The clinical tests used to diagnose this condition are Barlow's and Ortolani's.

15. Regarding the urethra
B only
The urethra consists of three parts. These are the prostatic, membranous and bulbar urethra. The membranous part is narrow and least dilatable. The bulbar urethra is inclined at 90° to the membranous urethra; an important fact to remember when passing instruments and catheters per urethra. There is no urethral artery; instead the urethra receives its blood supply from arteries to adjacent structures.

16. The following features are more common in ulcerative colitis than Crohn's disease

All false

Crohn's disease tends to cause more pain and weight loss than ulcerative colitis.

Ulcerative colitis always starts in the rectum and spreads more proximally in a continuous fashion affecting the terminal ileum in about 10% of cases (backwash ileitis). It mainly affects the mucosa.

17. The abdominal aorta

B, C, F, G

The aorta enters the abdomen at the level of T12 and bifurcates at the level of L4. It is the origin of the inferior mesenteric artery that lies posterior to the 3rd part of the duodenum.

18. The knee joint

A, B, E

The menisci, like other cartilagenous rims of synovial joints (i.e. shoulder and hip), are made of fibrocartilage.

19. The following are recognised complications of varicose veins

A, C, D, F

Varicose veins do not tend to fistulate.

20. Epiglottitis

A, E

This condition predominantly affects children aged 5–7 years. The most frequently encountered organism is *Haemophilus influenzae*. Airway obstruction can be a sudden and disastrous event and therefore senior anaesthetic help should be summoned to secure an airway. Unnecessary examination and investigation may jeopardize the patient's safety.

21. The systemic vascular resistance (SVR)

A, B, E

The factor that influences SVR more than any other factor is the diameter of the arterioles. During exercise the flow to the muscle increases and the SVR drops, thus maintaining a constant blood pressure.

The cardiac output is equal through both sides of the heart but the systemic pressure is much higher than the pulmonary pressure. This difference is due to a discrepancy in vascular resistance.

22. Tennis elbow

B, C

This condition results from tear and repair of the common extensor tendon which originates from the lateral epicondyle. There is usually pain and tenderness over this area but no swelling. Operative treatment is by detachment of the common extensor tendon.

23. The subclavian artery
A, B, D

The subclavian supplies the thyroid through its inferior thyroid branch. The superior thyroid artery is a branch of the external carotid artery. The right subclavian is a branch of the brachiocephalic artery.

24. Epistaxis
A, B, D, E

Bleeding in the older patient is more likely to be posterior and arterial in origin.

25. The factors which determine when an arterial stenosis becomes critical include
All true

A critical stenosis is a point at which further reduction of the radius produces a precipitous pressure drop across the stenosis. This occurs because of the exponential relation between the radius of the stenosis and the pressure gradient across it.

The pressure drop is determined by the degree of stenosis, i.e. the section area of the stenosis or its radius, which can be used to calculate the section area. High blood flow with greater run off produces a marked drop in pressure; therefore, a lesion will appear critical at a less severe stenosis than in a low-flow system. This explains claudication on exercise as this reduces the vascular resistance, therefore increasing run off. Exercise also increases flow which leads to a further drop in pressure across the stenosis. All this causes a lesion to appear critical without necessarily changing its radius.

26. Regarding calcium metabolism
A, C, E

Calcitonin is produced by the 'c' cells of the thyroid, in response to a state of hypercalcaemia, and will inhibit bone resorption and possibly intestinal absorption of calcium in an attempt to revert to normocalcaemia. Parathyroid hormone, responding to hypocalcaemia, increases bone resorption, calcium resorption from the kidneys and the conversion of vitamin D from 25-(OH)-D to 1, 25-(OH)2-D. Activated vitamin D increases intestinal absorption of calcium in addition to the actions of PTH.

27. Fluid management in the neonate
B, C, E

The gut is underdeveloped in the neonate and absorption is less effective than in adults.

28. The anatomical snuff box
A, B, D

The scaphoid and trapezium form most of the floor. The cutaneous nerve that passes here and supplies the skin of the snuff box is a branch of the radial nerve.

29. Popliteal artery aneurysms
A only

Popliteal artery aneurysms account for 70% of peripheral aneurysms. These are bilateral in 50% of cases and most commonly present with distal ischaemia. Repetitive trauma used to be the most frequent cause, encountered especially in cavalrymen, but atherosclerosis accounts for most cases now.

30. Carpal tunnel syndrome
A, C
Carpal tunnel syndrome occurs more commonly in females. The sensory deficit affects the palmar aspect of the thumb, index finger, middle finger and the lateral half of the ring finger. The condition should be treated conservatively when it occurs during pregnancy.

31. Jaundice in infants can be caused by
A, C, D, E
Hirschsprung's disease is congenital aganglionosis of the distal colon and rectum.

32. The spermatic cord contains
A, C, D, E, F
The only other constituent being lymphatics mainly from the testis.

33. Achalasia of the cardia
B, E
Achalasia usually presents in young adulthood and middle age. It is associated with squamous cell carcinoma of the middle third of the oesophagus. The condition is usually treated with endoscopic dilatation or a Heller's cardiomyotomy.

34. The following are complications of Billroth II gastrectomy
A, C, D, E
Billroth II gastrectomy is usually complicated by reduced food intake and mal-absorption. This results in weight loss, anaemia, steatorrhoea and various deficiencies.

35. Meckel's diverticulum
B, C, D
This is a true diverticulum which is a remnant of the vitelline duct. The commonest complications of Meckel's diverticulum are obstruction, intussusception and inflammation.

36. Renal cell carcinoma
A, B, C, D
Nephrectomy is not suitable for patients with metastases as the operative mortality is much higher than for patients with localized disease. Renal cell carcinoma is relatively resistant to chemotherapy. Radiotherapy is the best modality to palliate bone pain.

37. Osteoarthritis
B, D
Osteoarthritis is divided into primary and secondary. Primary osteoarthritis occurs in the absence of predisposing factors. Other X-ray changes are subchondral sclerosis, bone cysts and osteophytes. Realignment osteotomy can be used when only a part of the joint is involved.

38. The oesophagus
B, D

The oesophagus enters the abdominal cavity at the level of T10. It is covered by peritoneum for a short segment inside the abdomen where the anterior vagal nerve is closely applied to it.

39. Arterial wall structure
A, C, D

The aorta has a high elastin content which produces recoil in diastole. This converts potential energy into kinetic energy which maintains blood flow during diastole. The elastin content reduces with age producing stiffer arteries.

40. The submandibular salivary gland
A, B, D, E

It is the lingual nerve that has this relation to the submandibular duct.

41. The following substrates are virtually completely reabsorbed from the proximal tubule of the kidney
A, E

Only 67% of Na, Cl, K and water are reabsorbed in the proximal tubule.

42. Primary malignancies associated with secondary deposits in the adrenal gland include
All true

Secondary deposits in the adrenals are relatively rare accounting for only 10% of all adrenal malignancies.

43. Renal anatomy
B, C, E

The kidneys lie opposite the first to the third lumbar vertebrae. Their hila are at the level of the transpyloric plane, the left being slightly above and the right slightly below it. The left renal vein drains the left testis and the left suprarenal gland and passes in front of the abdominal aorta below the origin of the superior mesenteric artery before terminating in the inferior vena cava.

44. Acute renal infection
B, C, D

Pyonephrosis, i.e. collection of pus in the renal pelvis of an obstructed kidney, requires urgent radiological drainage to prevent total destruction of the kidney. Surgical drainage is employed in patients when medical therapy and radiologically placed drains fail to treat a carbuncle. Most cases of acute infections result from ascending organisms except in renal carbuncles when infection is spread via the haematogenous route, usually from a skin lesion.

45. Hydrocele
D only

Hydrocele is a collection of fluid between the tunica albuginea and tunica vaginalis. Primary hydrocele occurs in the absence of underlying pathology whereas a secondary hydrocele results from a pathological process, mainly affecting the testis, regardless of its nature. Treatment of secondary hydrocele is aimed at the primary pathology.

46. The following are radiological features of Colles' fracture
B, D

In Colles' fracture there is impaction, dorsal tilt and shift, and radial tilt and shift.

47. Carotid artery stenosis
B, D

Only about 20% of ischaemic strokes are caused by carotid artery stenosis. Duplex scanning and IV DSA are usually employed to investigate this condition. Selective carotid angiography carries the risk of dislodging atheroma. The risk of CVA following endarterectomy is about 1–4%.

48. Osteomalacia
A, D

Osteomalacia occurs in patients with vitamin D deficiency. This can be due to reduced intake, lack of exposure to sunlight or defective metabolism. The serum calcium is usually within normal limits.

49. Conn's syndrome
A, C, D, E

This condition is caused by an adrenocortical adenoma. The salient features are hyperaldosteronism, hypertension, hypokalaemia and low serum renin level. The treatment of choice is unilateral adrenalectomy.

50. The following are recognized complications of laparoscopic surgery
B, D, E

There is a significant reduction in the stress response to surgery and quicker recovery following laparoscopic surgery. However, absorption of carbon dioxide from the peritoneal cavity and splinting of the diaphragm cause hypercapnia.

EMQs

Theme: Shoulder conditions

61-c Posterior dislocation also occurs after electric shock. It should always be suspected in these two groups of patients when they complain of shoulder pain.

62-d

63-e Also known as impingement syndrome, painful arc and supraspinatus tendinitis.

Theme: Chronic limb ischaemia

64-g The degree of pathology and poor expectations preclude other treatment.

65-h The patient should be encouraged to stop smoking and to exercise.

66-b The severity of the symptoms and the nature of the atherosclerotic lesion make femoropopliteal bypass most appropriate.

Theme: Conditions that cause splenomegaly

67-f Travel to areas with a high prevalence of malaria should raise suspicion. A thick blood film will make the diagnosis.

68-d This condition presents as described in patients 30–50 years of age. Splenic tenderness is due to infarcts. Hodgkin's disease presents in a similar fashion but lymphadenopathy, especially of the cervical nodes, predominates.

69-a Alcoholism is a common cause of liver cirrhosis and portal hypertension. The haematemesis is likely to be secondary to oesophageal varices.

Theme: Ear and throat conditions

70-f Otitis media is a common infection of childhood. The condition is painful until the ear drum perforates. The condition responds to broad-spectrum antibiotics.

71-b This condition is very rare in the West now. The consequences are severe; therefore ENT opinion must be sought urgently.

72-a The diagnosis is made by examining the tonsils.

Theme: Cervical lymphadenopathy

73-c This is a typical presentation of nasopharyngeal malignancy which is common in Chinese people.

74-g Carcinomas of the tip of the tongue and the lower lip metastasize to the submental nodes.

75-e Any visceral malignancy can metastasize to the left supraclavicular node. Testicular malignancies usually spread to the para-aortic nodes.

76-f This will ultimately drain into the deep cervical nodes.

Theme: Aortoiliac atherosclerosis

77-d This patient is high risk due to his poor physical condition. An axillobifemoral bypass is much less of an undertaking than an aortobifemoral bypass. The diffuse nature of his disease makes it less suitable for non-surgical treatment.

78-a This short lesion seems ideal for angioplasty ± endovascular stent.

79-c The diffuse nature of the disease precludes interventional techniques. His symptoms warrant an operation and he is fit for aortobifemoral bypass.

Theme: Hoarse voice

80-d Persistent hoarse voice in the absence of any other obvious cause especially in smokers, is considered to be laryngeal carcinoma until proven otherwise.

81-g Bronchial carcinoma, especially on the left side, can invade the recurrent laryngeal nerve and cause hoarseness.

Theme: Bone 'tumours'

82-d Bone cysts are not tumours. They usually present in prepubertal children and mainly occur in the proximal ends of the humerus, femur and tibia.

83-b Ewing's sarcoma should be strongly suspected in any young patient with similar findings.

84-e Osteosarcoma is a recognized complication of Paget's disease. This is a fairly typical clinical picture.

Theme: Causes of right iliac fossa pain

85-c

86-h

87-b The urinary βhCG pregnancy test can be negative in tubal pregnancy.

Theme: Abdominal distension

88-c A delayed presentation of perforated duodenal ulcer.

89-e The pathophysiology of this condition is not clear. It is difficult to differentiate from mechanical obstruction but operative treatment is avoided if possible.

90-f The sigmoid colon is the commonest site for colonic volvulus. An attempt should be made to treat this condition by passing a flatus tube. Urgent surgery should be performed if this fails. This usually entails resection of the sigmoid and exteriorizing the bowel ends.

Theme: Carcinoma of the bladder

91-e The transurethral resection of the bladder tumour at the staging cystoscopy should be sufficient. The patient should be followed up with repeat cystoscopy.

92-b Although this stage of the disease can be treated with radical cystectomy, this man's poor general condition leaves him little choice but radiotherapy.

93-c Local chemotherapy or cystectomy are the options here. Chemotherapy is less of an undertaking to start with.

Theme: Vomiting

94-a The small bowel has herniated through the defect in the linea alba which was not closed adequately after laparoscopy.

95-d The vomiting is usually projectile. The stomach is dilated and there is a succussion splash. Serum chemistry and blood gases usually show alkalosis, hypokalaemia, hyponatraemia and dehydration.

Theme: Treatment of conditions of the thyroid

96-d This is the treatment undertaken by most surgeons for extrathyroid papillary carcinoma. The lymph nodes are removed when they are thought to be involved or in a modified block.

97-c A second course of medical treatment is unlikely to be effective. Her plans to become pregnant and have children preclude the use of radioiodine. Surgery is indicated in those under the age of 30, patients who refuse radioiodine and pregnant women or those planning pregnancy in the next 4 years.

98-b This patient has become hypothyroid and therefore thyroxine replacement is indicated. The patient is given a starting dose of 100 μg which is followed by adjustment according to TSH and free T4 levels. The incidence of hypothyroidism is reported to be between 10% and 50% following subtotal thyroidectomy.

Theme: Scrotal conditions in adults

99-b The inability to get above the swelling makes it inguinal in origin. The most likely diagnosis is a hernia.

100-d This is most likely to be a teratoma. Testicular tumours usually present with local symptoms, i.e. swelling or tenderness or both. Minor trauma may attract the patient's attention to the abnormality.

101-e This is more likely on the left as a result of the difference in venous anatomy between the right and left testis.

102-a When these contain spermatozoa they are called spermatocele. Epididymal cysts transilluminate brilliantly.

Theme: Fractured neck of femur

103-b The displaced head is likely to undergo avascular necrosis. It is removed at surgery and replaced with a prosthesis.

104-e Younger patients who are in reasonable health are best treated with a bipolar prosthesis or total hip replacement if the head has to be excised.

105-c

PRACTICE PAPER TWO: SYSTEM MODULES

MCQs

1. Malignant tumours of the thyroid gland

A   Papillary tumours commonly metastasize via the blood stream
B   Follicular carcinoma metastasizing to cervical lymph nodes used to be called lateral aberrant thyroid
C   Follicular carcinoma is diagnosed using FNAC
D   Lymphoma of the thyroid is associated with Hashimoto's thyroiditis
E   Anaplastic tumours are commonest in areas of endemic goitre

2. Rheumatoid arthritis

A   Is diagnosed by measuring rheumatoid factor titres
B   Infrequently affects the hands
C   Is an asymmetrical polyarthropathy
D   Is characterized by loss of joint space and juxta-articular erosions
E   Is a systemic disease affecting other tissues and organs

3. Cerebral perfusion and blood flow can be assessed with

A   PET
B   Magnetic resonance angiography
C   Duplex scanning
D   CT
E   The Fick principle using nitrous oxide

4. Bladder outflow obstruction

A   Can be caused by urethral valves
B   Is called functional when secondary to detrusor–sphincter dyssynergia
C   Can result in diverticula
D   The detrusor becomes thin and distended
E   Retained urine is liable to infection

5.   **Fissure-in-ano**

A   Occurs in the midline anteriorly in 70% of females
B   Can be treated with GTN ointment when acute
C   Is associated with Crohn's disease when it occurs posteriorly
D   Lateral external sphincterotomy is the operation of choice
E   Occurs more commonly in females

6.   **Regarding hydocele in children**

A   The sac of a congenital hydrocele communicates with the peritoneal cavity
B   Infantile hydrocele does not communicate with the peritoneal cavity
C   The size of congenital hydrocele varies with posture
D   It predisposes to testicular carcinoma
E   It predisposes to epididymal cysts

7.   **The following muscles form the rotator cuff**

A   Teres major
B   Supraspinatus
C   Latissmus dorsi
D   Rhomboid minor
E   Teres minor
F   Infraspinatus
G   Subscapularis

8.   **The following parameters are used to calculate GFR using inulin**

A   Serum concentration of inulin
B   Urine osmolality
C   Urinary inulin concentration
D   Urinary volume
E   Molecular weight of inulin

9.   **Regarding laparoscopic cholecystectomy**

A   A rising pressure gauge with little flow during the establishment of
    pneumoperitoneum indicates misplacement of the Verres needle
B   It carries an increased risk of bile duct injury
C   It is contraindicated in the presence of coagulopathy
D   It should not be performed if the patient has a history of previous abdominal
    surgery

10. The diaphragm

A   Its motor supply is mainly by C4
B   Develops from the septum transversum, the pleuroperitoneal membranes and the mesoderm of the posterior body wall
C   The commonest type of congenital diaphragmatic hernia is through the incompletely developed left pleuroperitoneal membrane
D   A congenital hernia may displace the apex beat
E   The left phrenic nerve passes through the oesophageal opening

11. Dupuytren's contractures are associated with the following

A   Alcoholic liver disease
B   Congenital cyanotic heart disease
C   Long-term phenytoin use
D   AIDS
E   Diabetes

12. Otitis media

A   Is rarely painful
B   A purulent discharge indicates perforation of the ear drum
C   *Klebsiella* is the commonest bacterial pathogen isolated
D   May be complicated by facial nerve palsy

13. The following factors are associated with varicose veins

A   Female sex
B   Deep venous thrombosis
C   Strong family history
D   Young age
E   Parity

14. Hand changes seen in rheumatoid arthritis include

A   Swan neck deformity
B   Boutonniere deformity
C   Dropped fingers
D   Metacarpophalangeal joint subluxation

15. **Blood flow**

A   Is proportional to the blood pressure
B   Is higher if the diameter of the conduit is larger
C   Is inversely proportional to the length of the conduit
D   Increases when the viscosity drops
E   Viscosity is lowest in the aorta

16. **The following factors favourably influence the long-term patency of a bypass graft**

A   Giving up smoking
B   The use of prosthetic grafts
C   The level of the graft; the more distal the better
D   The presence of confounding respiratory pathology
E   A good distal run off

17. **Regarding thyroxine**

A   Thyroxine (T4) is less efficacious than T3
B   T3 has a longer half-life than T4
C   T4 and TSH are integrated in a positive feedback loop
D   T3 and T4 are bound to thyroglobulin in plasma
E   Oral supplement with T3 requires tds dosing

18. **Carcinoma of the bladder**

A   Is always 'squamous cell' in type
B   Is a complication of bladder diverticulum
C   Is more common in smokers
D   May have an ulcerating appearance macroscopically
E   Is associated with schistosomiasis

19. **Fractures of the scaphoid**

A   Are most common in childhood
B   Frequently require open reduction
C   Usually occur across the proximal pole
D   Can be complicated by avascular necrosis of the distal fragment
E   Are readily detected on X-ray

20. Complications of atheroma

A   Embolization
B   Neoplasia
C   Thrombus formation
D   Metastatic calcification
E   Vessel occlusion

21. The following are recognized complications of transurethral resection of the prostate

A   TURP syndrome
B   Incontinence
C   Urethral stricture
D   Neoplastic change
E   Septicaemia
F   Hydrocele
G   Reactionary haemorrhage

22. The following diagnostic modalities are used to identify the site of active lower gastrointestinal haemorrhage

A   Colonoscopy
B   Barium enema
C   Nuclear medicine imaging
D   CT
E   Angiography

23. The following are recognized complications of hernias

A   Rupture
B   Perforation and abscess formation
C   Reduction en masse
D   Pregnancy in the hernial sac
E   Association with cholecystitis
F   Mesothelial hyperplasia

24. Flexor compartment of the forearm

A   The superficial group of muscles arise by a common origin from the medial epicondyle of the humerus
B   The main motor nerve supply is the ulnar nerve

C   The most superficial tendon is that of palmaris longus
D   The deep group can flex both the wrist and elbow
E   The ulnar and median nerves course through this compartment

25. **Complications of urethral stricture include**

A   Proximal stone formation
B   Bladder diverticulum
C   Hydronephrosis
D   Carcinoma of the penis
E   Paraurethral abscess

26. **Gastro-oesophageal reflux**

A   Occurs in most patients with hiatus hernia
B   Is associated with scleroderma
C   Can be confidently diagnosed in the absence of endoscopic changes
D   Can present with a clinical picture suggestive of asthma
E   Can produce dysplastic change in the epithelium of the lower third of the
    oesophagus known as 'Barrett's oesophagus'

27. **Maldescent of the testis**

A   Is more common in the premature neonate
B   The condition is called 'ectopic testis' if the testis is in the inguinal canal
C   Is associated with testicular malignancy
D   Can be diagnosed using laparoscopy

28. **Parotid neoplasms**

A   Are mostly malignant
B   Characteristically cause facial nerve palsy
C   Are most frequently pleomorphic adenomas
D   May present with Frey's syndrome
E   Surgery may be complicated by salivary duct fistulae
F   The facial nerve must be sacrificed in surgical excision of a deep pleomorphic
    adenoma

29. **Avascular necrosis of the femoral head is associated with**

A   Sickle cell disease
B   Prolonged steroid therapy

C Displaced subcapital fracture
D Alcoholism
E Deep sea diving

30. The popliteal fossa

A Is bounded by the two heads of gastrocnemius inferiorly
B Plantaris forms the floor of the fossa
C The popliteal vein is the deepest structure lying against the knee capsule
D Semi-membranosus and semi-tendinosus muscles form the upper lateral border
E Is bounded laterally by biceps femoris

31. Repair of arterial injury

A Can be performed using end-to-end anastomosis if enough length is available
B A braided absorbable suture is adequate for suturing a vein patch repair
C Vein grafts should not be used in trauma cases
D An arteriovenous fistula always requires surgery

32. The long saphenous vein

A Terminates at the saphenofemoral junction just below the midinguinal point
B Passes about a hand's breadth behind the medial border of the patella
C Communicates with the deep veins of the lower limb
D Passes behind the lateral malleolus
E Is closely related to the common peroneal nerve below the knee
F Has one tributary in the groin

33. Cushing's syndrome

A Is called Cushing's disease when the cause is an adrenal adenoma
B Is commonly caused by ectopic ACTH production
C Can be diagnosed using the short ACTH stimulation test
D Patients with this condition have a higher incidence of wound dehiscence
E Results in osteoporosis

34. Small bowel infarction

A May occur secondary to mesenteric venous thrombosis
B Is a recognized complication of myocardial infarction
C Is associated with a mortality rate of 30%

D   Abdominal X-ray may reveal gas in the bowel wall

E   May present with signs of intestinal obstruction

35. In the carpus

A   The scaphoid lies radially

B   The capitate lies between the scaphoid radially and the pisiform on the ulnar side

C   The hamate articulates with the first (thumb) metacarpal

D   The scaphoid is the most frequently fractured bone

E   The carpal tunnel is roofed by the extensor retinaculum

36. Aneurysms

A   Occur most commonly in the abdominal segment of the aorta

B   Of the abdominal aorta are more common in females

C   Of the femoral artery are more common than those of the popliteal artery

D   Are termed pseudoaneurysms when they mimic other pathology

37. Regarding the membranous layer of the superficial fascia covering the urogenital triangle

A   It is continuous with the superficial fascia of the abdominal wall

B   It is attached to the iliopectineal line laterally

C   It fuses with the fascia lata of the thigh

D   It encloses a space called the deep perineal pouch

E   Posteriorly it is attached to the perineal membrane

38. Large bowel obstruction

A   Occurs secondary to volvulus as the most common cause in the UK

B   Abdominal X-ray shows small bowel dilatation in 40% of cases

C   In the absence of mechanical cause is called paralytic ileus

D   Is accompanied by considerable fluid and electrolyte disturbance

39. With regard to the anterior abdominal wall

A   It derives its sensory supply from segments T7 to L1

B   The neurovascular bundles run between the external and internal oblique muscles

C   The transversus abdominis forms the posterior rectus sheath throughout the length of the recti

D   The venous drainage is to the inferior vena cava

40. **Nerve supply to the upper limb**

A   C5 dermatome is found on the lateral aspect of the forearm
B   Loss of C5 motor supply leads to inability to abduct the arm
C   The median nerve is the sensory supply to the palmar aspect of the lateral three and a half digits
D   The small muscles of the hand are supplied by C8 and T1
E   The musculocutaneous nerve supplies the flexor compartment of the arm

41. **Congenital renal abnormalities**

A   Include megaureter
B   Predispose to recurrent urinary tract infections
C   Polycystic disease of the kidney results in hypertension
D   Horseshoe kidney lies just below the superior mesenteric artery
E   Pelviureteric junction obstruction can be treated by pyeloplasty

42. **Acute pancreatitis**

A   Cannot be diagnosed if the serum amylase is less than 500 iu/l
B   May be a presenting feature of carcinoma of the head of the pancreas
C   Can be associated with thrombophlebitis migrans
D   Is said to be severe when the serum amylase is greater than 2000 iu/l
E   Is a recognized complication of cardiac surgery

43. **Hepatomegaly with an irregular margin can be seen in**

A   Hepatocellular carcinoma
B   Early alcoholic cirrhosis
C   Amyloidosis
D   Right-sided heart failure
E   Polycystic disease
F   Viral hepatitis

44. **The following conditions cause facial nerve palsy with involvement of the forehead muscles**

A   Bell's palsy
B   Cerebrovascular accident
C   Otitis media
D   Acoustic neuroma
E   Otitis externa
F   Pleomorphic adenoma

45. Club foot

A   Is more frequently seen in girls
B   Soft tissue release and elongation is used in the majority of patients to prevent deformity
C   On examination the deformity can be easily corrected with gentle manipulation
D   Is bilateral in a third of cases

46. The following conditions must be differentiated from arterial claudication as a cause of leg pain

A   Venous varicosities
B   Spinal stenosis
C   Venous claudication in post-thrombotic limb
D   Arteriovenous malformations
E   Arthritic disorders

47. Raynaud's phenomenon

A   Raynaud's disease is a rare condition affecting 1 in 100 000 of the population
B   Raynaud's syndrome is frequently idiopathic
C   Is associated with scleroderma
D   Patients with an exacerbation can benefit from prostacyclin infusion
E   Raynaud's syndrome occurs more commonly in females

48. The thyroid gland

A   Receives some of its blood supply via the superior thyroid artery, a branch of the internal carotid artery
B   The thyroid ima artery, when present, is a branch of the right subclavian artery
C   Blood is drained inferiorly into the anterior jugular veins
D   Is supplied by the recurrent laryngeal nerve
E   The superior thyroid veins drain into the internal jugular veins
F   Is enclosed by the pretracheal fascia

49. The spleen

A   There is increased risk of serious infections due to encapsulated organisms in the asplenic patient
B   Is the most frequently injured organ in blunt abdominal trauma
C   Is supplied by the splenic artery which is a branch of the left gastric artery
D   The gastrosplenic ligament contains the tail of the pancreas and the splenic vessels
E   Can be enlarged in lymphoma

50. Carcinoma of the penis

A Is rare in those circumcised in infancy
B Is typically squamous
C Is associated with human papilloma virus infection
D Spreads to the external iliac lymph nodes
E Is associated with picornavirus infection

EMQs

Theme: Innervation of lower limb muscles

Options:
a Sural nerve
b Deep peroneal nerve
c Superficial peroneal nerve
d Tibial nerve
e Femoral nerve
f Saphenous nerve
g Obturator nerve

For each of the muscles below, choose the single most likely nerve from the list above.
Each option may be used once, more than once or not at all.

61. Quadriceps femoris
62. Tibialis anterior
63. Peroneus longus
64. Adductor magnus

Theme: Acute limb ischaemia

Options:
a Thrombolysis
b Vascular repair
c Thrombectomy
d Embolectomy
e Amputation
f Phenol sympathectomy
g Pain relief
h External fixation

For each of the case scenarios below, choose the single most likely option from the list
above. Each option may be used once, more than once or not at all.

65. A 19-year-old victim of an explosion injury presents with an ischaemic foot. There is loss of popliteal artery continuity and the distal end is difficult to find due to extensive soft tissue loss. The forefoot was amputated in the blast.

66. A 70-year-old woman with atrial fibrillation develops acute lower limb ischaemia. She was admitted 2 weeks earlier to a medical ward with a cerebrovascular accident. She has recovered most of her neurological deficit.

67. A 26-year-old builder fell off a scaffold from a height of 7 m. He has a compound fracture of the femur. His distal pulses vary with the position of his leg.

Theme: Thyrotoxicosis

Options:

a   Multinodular goitre
b   Hashimoto's thyroiditis
c   Grave's disease
d   Toxic adenoma
e   Thyroxine overdose
f   Thyroid lymphoma
g   Ovarian teratoma

For each of the case scenarios below, choose the single most likely option from the list above. Each option may be used once, more than once or not at all.

68. A 35-year-old female complains of excessive sweating, erratic menstrual period and diarrhoea. On examination she has a palpable lump on the right of the trachea. Thyroid function tests show elevated T3 and suppressed TSH. A nuclear medicine scan shows a solitary 'hot' nodule.

69. A 41-year-old female presents with 'bulging' eyes, weight loss and diarrhoea. On examination her thyroid is enlarged and the thyroid function tests show elevated T3 and T4 with undetectable TSH. The nuclear scan shows increased isotope uptake by the gland.

Theme: Diarrhoea

Options:

a   Cholera
b   Diverticular disease
c   Villous adenoma
d   Campylobacter food poisoning
e   Crohn's disease
f   Gluten intolerance
g   Irritable bowel syndrome
h   Appendicitis

For each of the case scenarios below, choose the single most likely option from the list above. Each option may be used once, more than once or not at all.

70. A 45-year-old woman complains of diarrhoea and colicky lower abdominal pain following ingestion of milk. A bird had picked at the bottle's foil cap.
71. A 7-year-old girl presents with diarrhoea and lower abdominal pain mainly in the right iliac fossa. Her temperature is 38°C.
72. A 62-year-old man is brought into A&E collapsed. He is incontinent of slimy diarrhoea.
73. A 72-year-old woman presents with a history of recurrent bouts of left iliac fossa pain and diarrhoea over the past couple of years.

Theme: Treatment of urological trauma

Options:
a   Urethral catheterization
b   Laparotomy
c   Ileal conduit
d   Suprapubic catheterization
e   Nephrectomy
f   Double J stent insertion
g   Observation
h   Cystoscopy

For each of the case scenarios below, choose the single most likely option from the list above. Each option may be used once, more than once or not at all.

74. An 18-year-old rider falls off her horse. In A&E the urine appears clear but dipstix reveals blood ($+ +$). An IVU is normal.
75. A motorcyclist presents at hospital following an accident. He has injuries to his perineum and blood at the urethral meatus. His bladder is palpable. Urethral catheterization is attempted but fails.
76. A 57-year-old man sustains a pelvic fracture following a road traffic accident. A cystogram reveals minor extraperitoneal urine extravasation.

Theme: Knee injuries

Options:
a   Medial ligament tear
b   Anterior cruciate ligament tear
c   Meniscal tear
d   Posterior cruciate ligament tear
e   Fractured patella
f   Dislocation of the patella
g   Osgood–Schlatter's disease

For each of the case scenarios below, choose the single most likely option from the list above. Each option may be used once, more than once or not at all.

77. Tom is 26 years old. He sustained a twisting injury to his right knee while playing football. The pain was severe enough that he had to stop playing. His knee is moderately swollen 12 hours later.
78. A 30-year-old man injured his knee while playing rugby. His right foot was stuck in the mud while the rest of his body rotated to the right. There was sudden pain and almost immediate swelling of the knee.
79. A 22-year-old woman collapsed while walking. On examination the knee joint is immobile and the medial femoral condyle is prominent.

Theme: Management of varicose veins

Options:
a   Compression stockings
b   Reassurance
c   Saphenofemoral junction ligation and stripping of the long saphenous vein
d   Injection sclerotherapy
e   Multiple avulsions
f   Excision of the ulcer and skin grafting
g   Subfascial endoscopic perforator vein ligation

For each of the case scenarios below, choose the single most likely option from the list above. Each option may be used once, more than once or not at all.

80. A 45-year-old male with a 2-year history of varicose veins presents with unsightly varicosities in the distribution of the right long saphenous vein. These cause an ache and swelling at the end of a long day at the office. He had deep vein thrombosis in the right leg 8 years ago and subsequent pulmonary embolus. Investigations reveal saphenofemoral incompetence.
81. A 56-year-old woman with a long-standing history of varicose veins complains of skin changes on her legs. On examination she has very thin skin above the medial malleolus. This is on the verge of ulcerating. She has saphenofemoral incompetence.
82. A 30-year-old woman presents with mild varicosities behind her left knee. She is anxious because her mother was admitted to hospital for 2 weeks when she had deep vein thrombosis and pulmonary embolus.
83. A 43-year-old woman presents with troublesome below knee varicose veins. On examination she has severe lipodermatosclerosis and there is no evidence of saphenopopliteal or saphenofemoral incompetence. The deep venous system appears normal.

Theme: Bilious vomiting in infants

Options:

a   Pyloric stenosis
b   Oesphageal atresia
c   Malrotation of the gut
d   Intussusception
e   Diaphragmatic hernia
f   Meconium ileus
g   Duodenal atresia

For each of the case scenarios below, choose the single most likely option from the list above. Each option may be used once, more than once or not at all.

84. An apparently healthy newborn baby was found to have a distended abdomen. The following day she developed bilious vomiting and 2 days later she had not opened her bowels. An X-ray of the abdomen reveals distended bowel loops.

85. A healthy 9-month-old boy presents with intermittent attacks of screaming and drawing up his knees. There is a palpable mass in the upper abdomen.

86. A newborn baby developed bilious vomiting a few hours after delivery. A plain abdominal X-ray shows a double bubble appearance.

Theme: Rectal bleeding

Options:

a   Diverticular disease
b   Angiodysplasia
c   Carcinoma of the colon
d   Colonic polyps
e   Ischaemic colitis
f   Haemorrhoids
g   Fissure-in-ano
h   Carcinoma of the anus

For each of the case scenarios below, choose the single most likely option from the list above. Each option may be used once, more than once or not at all.

87. A 63-year-old woman presents with recurrent attacks of dark rectal bleeding. She complained of an 18-month history of intermittent left iliac fossa pain and erratic bowel habit. There has been no weight loss.

88. A 23-year-old female presents with fresh bleeding on the toilet paper and pain on defaecation. A rectal examination was not possible to perform due to pain.

89. A 58-year-old man presents with three episodes of rectal bleeding. The blood is dark in colour and mixed with the stools. He also noticed slime on the toilet paper. There has been weight loss of half a stone.

Theme: Haematuria

Options:

a   Carcinoma of the prostate
b   Renal cell carcinoma
c   Transitional cell carcinoma
d   Schistosomiasis
e   Urinary tract infection
f   Benign prostatic hypertrophy
g   Ureteric colic

For each of the case scenarios below, choose the single most likely option from the list above. Each option may be used once, more than once or not at all.

90.   A 14 year old presents with macroscopic haematuria. He is an immigrant from Egypt.
91.   A 29-year-old salesman presents with pain in the right loin. The pain radiates to the scrotum. He has also noticed a red tinge to his urine.
92.   A 63-year-old woman presents with painless macroscopic haematuria. She has had no pain or urinary symptoms otherwise.

Theme: Innervation of the bladder

Options:

a   A transection of dorsal root of T10
b   Injury to sacral segments 1, 2 and 3
c   The obturator nerve
d   The greater splanchnic nerve
e   The external pudendal nerve
f   Spinal transection at the level of the 9th thoracic segment
g   L1, 2
h   Injury to sacral segments 2, 3 and 4

For each of the case scenarios below, choose the single most likely option from the list above. Each option may be used once, more than once or not at all.

93.   A 26-year-old man was involved in a road traffic accident a year ago. He now has a tendency to pass urine in a reflex fashion when the bladder is full and without any control.
94.   His friend was a passenger in the car. He has a palpable bladder and dribbles continuously.

Theme: Brachial plexus injuries

Options:
a   C6, 7, 8
b   C5
c   C5, 6
d   C5, 6, 7, 8 and T1
e   C7, 8 and T1
f   C8 and T1
g   C5, 6, 7

For each of the case scenarios below, choose the single most likely option from the list above. Each option may be used once, more than once or not at all.

95. Jennifer, a healthy 3.8 kg full-term baby, was born 5 hours ago after prolonged labour. Her mother is concerned as her right arm appears medially rotated with the palm of the hand facing backwards.

96. Mrs Payne is a 64-year-old woman who was a standing passenger on the underground. When the train made a sudden stop she clutched hold of the overhead railing to prevent herself from falling. The A&E officer finds weakness of the small muscles of the hand and sensory loss over the medial aspect of the hand and forearm.

97. A 24-year-old motorcyclist is brought to A&E by an ambulance having had a road traffic accident. He is found to be conscious with abrasions to his right shoulder and the right half of his face. The right upper limb is paralysed and insensate.

Theme: Facial nerve palsy

Options:
a   Cerebrovascular accident
b   Bell's palsy
c   Parotid malignancy
d   Ramsay Hunt syndrome (herpes zoster)
e   Acoustic neuroma
f   Chronic otitis media
g   Meningitis
h   Pleomorphic adenoma of the parotid gland

For each of the case scenarios below, choose the single most likely option from the list above. Each option may be used once, more than once or not at all.

98. A 55-year-old man presents with right facial paresis. On examination he appears to have lost the normal skin creases of the right forehead. He also has painful vesicles on the right external auditory meatus.

99. A 75-year-old woman complains of drooping of the left side of her face. On examination there is drooping of the angle of the mouth and sagging of the lower eyelid. There is also ipsilateral swelling over the angle of the jaw.

Theme: Groin swellings

Options:
a   Direct inguinal hernia
b   Indirect inguinal hernia
c   Femoral hernia
d   Undescended testis
e   Saphena varix
f   Iliofemoral aneurysm
g   Lymphogranuloma venereum

For each of the case scenarios below, choose the single most likely option from the list above. Each option may be used once, more than once or not at all.

100. An 18-year-old male presents with a 2-week history of progressively enlarging inguinal swelling which is constant, tender and fluctuant.
101. A 70-year-old woman with recent weight loss presents with a 3-day history of tender right groin swelling. There is marked skin erythema.
102. A 72-year-old man presents with a 6-month history of right groin swelling which descends into his scrotum. This disappears on lying flat.

Theme: Investigation of the renal tract

Options:
a   IVU
b   CT
c   Ultrasound Scan
d   MRI
e   Renal angiogram
f   Cystoscopy
g   Urethrography

For each of the case scenarios below, choose the single most likely option from the list above. Each option may be used once, more than once or not at all.

103. A 26-year-old man presents with loin pain and microscopic haematuria.
104. A 76-year-old female presents with pneumaturia.
105. An 18-year-old male involved in a road traffic accident presents with blood at the urethral meatus and urinary retention.

ANSWERS TO PRACTICE PAPER TWO

The letters of the correct answers are given

MCQs

1. Malignant tumours of the thyroid gland
D, E

Papillary carcinoma is a well-differentiated thyroid tumour. It characteristically metastasizes to the cervical lymph nodes. Involved nodes when biopsied appear replaced by the malignant thyroid tissue and used to be called 'lateral aberrant thyroid'.

Follicular carcinoma appears similar to follicular adenoma histologically except that the carcinoma invades the thyroid capsule. This invasion needs to be assessed on histology rather than cytology.

2. Rheumatoid arthritis
D, E

Rheumatoid factor is only positive in 80% of cases. The diagnosis is made by the finding of certain clinical features. The hand joints are most commonly affected in this condition of symmetrical polyarthropathy.

3. Cerebral perfusion and blood flow can be assessed with
A, B, C, E

CT is not used to measure cerebral blood flow. PET employs radiolabelled compounds to obtain physiological images of the brain.

4. Bladder outflow obstruction
A, B, C, E

Chronic retention also leads to detrusor hypertrophy and hydronephrosis.

5. Fissure-in-ano
B, E

Anal fissures occur in the midline posteriorly in most cases but more so in males than females. Crohn's disease should be suspected if the fissure occurs laterally. The preferred surgical treatment is internal sphincterotomy.

6. Regarding hydocele in children
A, B, C

A congenital (communicating) hydrocele is continuous with the peritoneal cavity. The size of the hydrocele is therefore variable with posture. In infantile hydrocele the processus vaginalis remains patent in the scrotum and cord but gets obliterated proximally, usually at the level of the deep inguinal ring.

7. **The following muscles form the rotator cuff**

B, E, F, G

8. **The following parameters are used to calculate GFR using inulin**

A, C, D

$$GFR = U_{in} \times V \div P_{in}$$

GFR, glomerular filtration rate; U_{in}, urinary inulin concentration; P_{in}, plasma inulin concentration; V, volume of urine.

9. **Regarding laparoscopic cholecystectomy**

A, B, C

Previous abdominal surgery is not an absolute contraindication.

10. **The diaphragm**

A, B, C, D

The left phrenic nerve pierces the diaphragm whereas the right passes through the caval opening.

11. **Dupuytren's contractures are associated with the following**

A, C, D, E

12. **Otitis media**

B, D

Pneumococcus, *Haemophilus* and *Streptococci* are the commonest infecting bacteria. This condition, which mostly affects young children, is quite painful until the tympanic membrane perforates. Facial nerve palsy is usually temporary and occurs secondary to involvement of the nerve as it passes through the middle ear.

13. **The following factors are associated with varicose veins**

A, B, C, E

Older rather than younger age is associated with varicose veins.

14. **Hand changes seen in rheumatoid arthritis include**

All true

15. **Blood flow**

A, B, C, D

Blood flow $= (\pi \times \Delta Pressure \times Radius^4) \div (8 \times Viscosity\ of\ blood \times Length)$

The length and radius are those of the conduit. The difference in pressure is between the two ends of the conduit. The relative viscosity of blood is lower in smaller arteries.

16. The following factors favourably influence the long-term patency of a bypass graft
A, E
Proximal grafts do better than distal ones. A vein graft has a higher patency rate at 5 years than a prosthetic graft.

17. Regarding thyroxine
A, E
T4 has a higher plasma concentration and longer half-life than T3. Both hormones are carried by thyroid-binding globulin in plasma. Thyroglobulin is present in the colloid and functions as a reservoir for T3 and T4. The secretion of T3 and T4 is regulated by the hypothalamus→pituitary→thyroid axis; T3 and T4 have a negative feedback effect on TRH and TSH release.

18. Carcinoma of the bladder
B, C, D, E
Some 90% of bladder tumours arise in transitional epithelium. Squamous cell carcinoma arises as a consequence of chronic inflammation, e.g. due to infestation by schistosomiasis, or in a bladder diverticulum.

19. Fractures of the scaphoid
D only
Fractures of the scaphoid are most commonly seen in young men.

20. Complications of atheroma
A, C, E
Neoplasia is not a recognized complication of atheroma. The pathological calcification of an atheromatous plaque is dystrophic, i.e. in the presence of normal serum calcium levels. Metastatic calcification occurs in pathological states of hypercalcaemia.

21. The following are recognized complications of transurethral resection of the prostate
A, B, C, E, G

22. The following diagnostic modalities are used to identify the site of active lower gastrointestinal haemorrhage
A, C, E
Colonoscopy can show the site of active bleeding although it is often unhelpful in practice. Barium enema can reveal carcinoma, diverticular disease and ischaemic bowel, but the source of the bleeding cannot be identified with certainty.

23. The following are recognized complications of hernias
A, B, C, D, F
Mesothelial hyperplasia can occur secondary to repeated bowel incarceration. Other complications include strangulation, involvement in peritoneal pathology, sliding hernia and testicular complications.

24. Flexor compartment of the forearm
A, C, E
The main motor supply is by the median nerve. The ulnar nerve supplies flexor carpi ulnaris and part of flexor digitorum profundus. The deep group of muscles originates from the radius, ulna and the interosseous membrane, therefore spanning the wrist only. The superficial group spans the elbow and wrist enabling them to flex both.

25. Complications of urethral stricture include
A, B, C, E
The complications are similar to those of prostatic obstruction. Chronic inflammation and calculi give rise to squamous cell carcinoma.

26. Gastro-oesophageal reflux
B, D
Only about a third of patients with hiatus hernia have symptomatic reflux. Upper gastrointestinal endoscopy fails to show signs of reflux in 30% of patients. Barrett's is a metaplastic change from squamous to columnar epithelium.

27. Maldescent of the testis
A, C, D
Ectopic testis exists if the testis is in a position which lies outside its normal route of descent from the retroperitoneum to the scrotum.

28. Parotid neoplasms
C, E
About 90% of parotid neoplasms are adenomas and 90% of these are pleomorphic. Facial nerve invasion is characteristic of malignant neoplasms. The facial nerve is carefully preserved in excision of pleomorphic adenoma of any depth. Frey's syndrome is gustatory sweating which is a complication of thyroidectomy.

29. Avascular necrosis of the femoral head is associated with
All true
Decompression illness in deep sea divers can result in avascular necrosis.

30. The popliteal fossa
A, E
This diamond-shaped fossa is bounded inferiorly by the two heads of gastrocnemius. The upper lateral border is formed by biceps femoris and the upper medial border by semi-membranosus and semi-tendinosus muscles. Popliteus covers part of the floor. The popliteal artery is the deepest structure lying close to the joint capsule. The tibial nerve is the most superficial.

31. Repair of arterial injury
A only

Vascular repairs require a synthetic non-absorbable suture material which is also a monofilament. Prolene™ is a good example. An interposition graft can be used when enough length for end-to-end anastomosis is not available. This can be either a length of vein or synthetic graft. An arteriovenous fistula can be treated by pressure using a Doppler probe.

32. The long saphenous vein
B, C

The long saphenous vein passes anterior to the medial malleolus and ascends on the medial aspect of the leg where it has the described relation to the knee. In this course it is closely associated with the saphenous nerve. In the groin, the vein is joined by a variable number of tributaries. These include the superficial circumflex iliac, the superficial epigastric and the superficial external pudendal veins. The saphenofemoral junction lies about 4 cm inferior and lateral to the pubic tubercle.

33. Cushing's syndrome
D, E

Cushing's disease is caused by a pituitary adenoma. The commonest cause of Cushing's syndrome is secondary to steroid therapy. Estimations of plasma and urinary cortisol levels and the dexamethasone suppression tests are used to diagnose the condition.

34. Small bowel infarction
A, B, D, E

Small bowel ischaemia may result from superior mesenteric artery atherosclerosis or thromboembolism, shock or mesenteric venous thrombosis. Most emboli arise from the heart secondary to either arrhythmia, valvular lesion or infarction. Acute bowel ischaemia carries a mortality of over 70%.

35. In the carpus
A, D

The carpus is composed of eight bones arranged in two rows. The proximal row contains the scaphoid, lunate, triquetral and pisiform from radial to ulnar. The distal row contains the trapezium, trapezoid, capitate and hamate from radial to medial.

36. Aneurysms
A

Abdominal aortic aneurysm has a prevalence of 1–4% in those over the age of 50 in the UK. Males are more frequently affected than females. The popliteal artery is the most commonly affected peripheral artery. True aneurysms are pathological dilatations of all layers of the wall, whereas in pseudoaneurysms not all the layers are involved.

37. Regarding the membranous layer of the superficial fascia covering the urogenital triangle
A, C, E
The lateral attachment of this fascial layer is to the ischiopubic rami. The space deep to this layer is called the superficial pouch. Extravasation of urine or blood from a ruptured urethra may fill this potential space and extend over the scrotum, penis and anterior abdominal wall. It does not track to the anal triangle posteriorly or the thighs laterally because of its attachments.

38. Large bowel obstruction
D
Carcinoma of the colon is the commonest cause in the UK. The iliocaecal valve is incompetent in about 10% of cases. In the absence of a mechanical cause the condition is known as pseudo-obstruction.

39. With regard to the anterior abdominal wall
A
The neurovascular bundle runs between the internal oblique and the transversus abdominis. The posterior rectus sheath terminates at the level of the arcuate line which is halfway between the umbilicus and the pubic symphysis. The superficial veins above the umbilicus drain to the superior vena cava and the area below the umbilicus drains to the inferior vena cava.

40. Nerve supply to the upper limb
B, C, D
The C5 dermatome is on the lateral aspect of the arm.

41. Congenital renal abnormalities
A, B, C, E
The kidneys are pelvic organs in the embryo. They ascend during development to their adult position. In 'horseshoe kidney' ascent is arrested below the lowest anterior branch of the aorta, i.e. the inferior mesenteric artery.

42. Acute pancreatitis
B, E
Amylase is not always markedly raised, especially in patients with delayed presentation.
Specific scores such as 'Ranson's' are used to gauge the severity of the attack. The degree of hyperamylasaemia is not one of the parameters used in these scores.
Thrombophlebitis migrans is associated with pancreatic carcinoma.

43. Hepatomegaly with an irregular margin can be seen in
A, E
The liver enlarges uniformly in early stages of alcoholic cirrhosis.

44. The following conditions cause facial nerve palsy with involvement of the forehead muscles

A, C, D

Upper motor neuron lesions (e.g. CVA) result in paralysis of the lower facial muscle only; the forehead has a dual supply. Benign tumours of the parotid do not invade the facial nerve.

45. Club foot

D only

This condition is more common in boys (2:1). Unlike postural talipes, the deformity is fixed and cannot be overcome with gentle manipulation. The mainstay of treatment is splinting. Operative treatment is only used in resistant cases.

46. The following conditions must be differentiated from arterial claudication as a cause of leg pain

B, C, E

Varicose veins can cause an ache but the pain is not usually mistaken for claudication.

47. Raynaud's phenomenon

C, D, E

Raynaud's disease affects 5–10% of young females (in their 30s) in temperate climates. The condition is termed Raynaud's disease when it occurs in young women with no obvious pathology predisposing to it. In the presence of a causative condition it is usually known as Raynaud's syndrome or phenomenon.

48. The thyroid gland

E, F

The thyroid is supplied by two pairs of arteries; the superior thyroid artery arises from the external carotid artery and the inferior thyroid from the subclavian artery. A third artery, the thyroid ima, is a variable artery which can arise from the arch of the aorta, the brachiocephalic or left common carotid arteries. The superior and middle pairs of veins drain blood into the internal jugular vein on each side. The inferior veins drain into the brachiocephalic veins.

49. The spleen

A, B, E

The splenic artery is a branch of the coeliac artery. It runs with the splenic vein and the tail of the pancreas to the splenic hilum in the lienorenal ligament.

50. Carcinoma of the penis

A, B, C

This is a rare condition which affects those over the age of 45. The lesion can be exophytic or ulcerated and the lymphatic spread is to the inguinal nodes. The condition is treated by amputation with a 5-year survival rate of about 70%.

EMQs

Theme: Innervation of lower limb muscles
61-e   The femoral nerve also innervates iliacus, pectineus and sartorius. Quadriceps
        femoris is composed of the three vastus muscles and rectus femoris.
62-b   The deep peroneal is also known as the anterior tibial nerve. It supplies the
        muscles of the anterior compartment of the leg, extensor hallucis longus,
        extensor digitorum longus, extensor digitorum brevis and peroneus tertius, in
        addition to tibialis anterior.
63-c   It also supplies peroneus brevis.
64-g   The obturator nerve supplies the muscles of the medial compartment of the thigh.

Theme: Acute ischaemia
65-e   The degree of injury is not compatible with reconstruction.
66-d   A recent cerebrovascular accident is a contraindication to thrombolysis.
67-h   External fixation may be all that is required to maintain vascular supply
        distally.

Theme: Thyrotoxicosis
68-d   This condition is found in females in about 90% of cases. The excessive
        hormone can be either T3 or T4. The eyes are not usually involved.
69-c   The findings described and the presence of thyroid-stimulating
        immunoglobulins are characteristic of this condition. The eyes are frequently
        involved.

Theme: Diarrhoea
70-d   Campylobacters are a common cause of gastroenteritis in man. They are
        carried by a variety of birds and animals.
71-h
72-c   Production of copious amounts of potassium-rich mucus by a villous adenoma
        can cause severe dehydration and electrolyte imbalance.
73-b

Theme: Treatment of urological trauma
74-g   Most minor renal trauma can be managed conservatively.
75-d   This patient is considered to have a transected urethra until proven otherwise.
76-a   Urethral catheterization is the treatment of choice for minor injuries of this type.

Theme: Knee injuries
77-c
78-b   Both meniscal tear and cruciate ligament injury can result from rotational and
        lateral violence. The timing of the swelling is one of the distinguishing factors.
79-f   This condition occurs more commonly in females and is frequently bilateral.
        Conservative treatment by strengthening the quadriceps is advised. Recurrence of
        symptoms and failure of conservative treatment call for operative intervention.

Theme: Management of varicose veins

80-a Deep vein thrombosis results in destruction of the valves. This patient's symptoms and the fact that he had a previous thrombosis preclude surgical treatment. Graded compression stockings should help control his symptoms.

81-c This woman will develop troublesome ulceration if surgery is not performed urgently.

82-b Counselling and reassurance are all that is required. The patient should be told that there is no association between varicose veins and pulmonary embolus.

83-g Again, there is a danger of venous ulceration and surgery is indicated. Perforator incompetence is the cause of this patient's symptoms.

Theme: Bilious vomiting in infants

84-f Meconium ileus occurs in about 15% of babies born with cystic fibrosis, an autosomal recessive condition which affects about 1 in 2000 babies. The rectum is usually empty and the colon is collapsed. Gastrografin enema carried out as an investigation can sometimes be therapeutic.

85-d This condition occurs most commonly under the age of 1 and in boys. The typical 'redcurrant jelly' faeces occurs within about 24 hours of the onset of the condition.

86-g This condition has an incidence of about 1 in 6000. It is associated with other abnormalities especially Down's syndrome and congenital heart disease.

Theme: Rectal bleeding

87-a All the features and the chronicity of the symptoms suggest diverticular disease.

88-g Sphincter spasm causes digital examination to be very painful. This is not necessary as the fissure will be seen without the need for rectal examination.

89-c This is considered to be carcinoma of the colon until proven otherwise.

Theme: Haematuria

90-d Egypt is one of the areas with a high incidence of schistosomiasis.

91-g

92-c This is the most likely cause. Urine cytology, an IVU and cystoscopy should reveal the source of bleeding.

Theme: Innervation of the bladder

93-f The injury is suprasacral. This results in 'automatic reflex bladder'.

94-h Loss of sacral innervation results in atonic detrusor, and consequently the patient develops retention and overflow incontinence.

Theme: Brachial plexus injuries

95-c This is Erb's palsy.

96-f This is Dejerine–Klumpke palsy which usually gives the typical appearance of claw hand. It can also be associated with Horner's syndrome if the cervical sympathetic ganglia are involved.

97-d This patient has lost all innervation to his right upper limb.

Theme: Facial nerve palsy

98-d Involvement of the muscles of the forehead indicates a lower motor neuron lesion. The painful vesicles on the external auditory meatus point to this diagnosis. This condition occurs in the elderly and the immunologically compromised.

99-c The position of the swelling is compatible with parotid pathology. Malignant tumours of the parotid tend to invade the facial nerve (unlike pleomorphic adenoma).

Theme: Groin swellings

100-g This is a sexually transmitted infection caused by *Chlamydia trachomatis*.

101-c

102-b Indirect inguinal hernias tend to descend into the scrotum.

Theme: Investigation of the renal tract

103-a The history is compatible with ureteric colic. An IVU including a plain control film is the appropriate investigation.

104-f Cystoscopy will help identify the site of the fistula.

105-g The findings are consistent with urethral injury. A contrast study will delineate the site of injury.

PRACTICE PAPER THREE: SYSTEM MODULES

MCQs

1. Regarding muscles that act on the fingers

A Flexor digitorum superficialis flexes the metacarpophalangeal and proximal interphalangeal joints

B The lumbricals of the index and middle fingers are supplied by the radial nerve

C The muscles of the extensor compartment of the forearm are supplied by the radial nerve and its motor branches

D Extensor indicis can be used to replace a ruptured extensor pollicis longus

E Flexor digitorum profundus flexes the distal interphalangeal joints

2. The femoral triangle

A Is bounded medially by the medial border of adductor longus

B Iliacus, psoas and pectineus form the floor of the triangle

C The lateral limit is the medial border of sartorius

D The femoral nerve is the most lateral of the neurovascular bundle in the triangle

E The femoral canal accommodates the femoral vein when distended

3. Clinical diagnosis of varicose veins

A The detection of a venous thrill on coughing while palpating the long aspenous vein in the groin indicates midthigh perforator incompetence

B Inability to fill the varicosities after the application of a tourniquet above the midthigh is a sign of saphenofemoral incompetence

C The presence of ulceration above the lateral malleolus is a proof of chronic varicose veins

D The distribution of varicosities is a good indicator of whether the condition is secondary to perforator incompetence

E Reflux is indicated by a biphasic Doppler signal when squeezing the patient's calf

4.   Complications of pancreatitis

A   ARDS is characterized by hypoxia, poor lung compliance and increased left atrial pressure
B   Pseudocysts less than 6 cm in diameter can be treated conservatively
C   Pseudocysts may be treated with endoscopic drainage
D   Renal failure can be prevented with fluid restriction

5.   Renal trauma

A   Occurs more commonly in kidneys with congenital abnormalities
B   May be associated with paralytic ileus
C   Minor injuries should be treated conservatively
D   Is often secondary to blunt trauma
E   May result in long-term hypertension

6.   The cubital fossa

A   Brachialis forms the floor of the fossa
B   Pronator teres is the lateral boundary
C   The brachial artery lies medial to the tendon of biceps
D   The brachial artery lies lateral to the ulnar nerve
E   The roof is formed by the deep fascia which is reinforced by the bicipital aponeurosis medially

7.   The thoracic inlet

A   The subclavian artery passes behind the scalenus medius muscle
B   The T1 root of the brachial plexus passes into the axilla under the 1st rib
C   The subclavian vessels and brachial plexus are covered by the axillary sheath as they pass from the root of the neck to the axilla
D   The thoracic duct enters the venous system at the junction of the left internal jugular and subclavian vein
E   The brachial plexus is composed of three trunks as it passes over the 1st rib
F   The stellate ganglion, formed by the fusion of the inferior cervical and 1st thoracic ganglia, lies on the neck of the 1st rib

8.   Phaeochromocytoma

A   Is frequently bilateral
B   Is characteristically malignant

C Can be diagnosed by estimating plasma cortisol level
D Surgery can be complicated by hypertensive crisis
E Surgery should be preceded by a course of α and β blockers

9. Gastric acid secretion is stimulated by

A Histamine
B Noradrenaline
C Gastrin
D Prostaglandin
E Acetylcholine
F Phrenic nerve

10. Urodynamic studies

A Compliance is a description of change in intravesical pressure as the bladder volume changes
B Low compliance is observed in interstitial cystitis
C The detrusor pressure is the intravesical pressure subtracted from the rectal pressure
D Uroflowmetry only measures the urinary flow rate

11. Paget's disease of the bone

A Is common in Africa
B Is associated with osteosarcoma of the bone
C Patients have elevated serum calcium, phosphate and alkaline phosphatase
D May cause deafness
E The bone is brittle despite cortical thickening

12. Surface anatomy of some palpable pulses

A The femoral artery is palpable 4 cm inferolateral to the pubic tubercle
B The brachial artery is palpable lateral to the tendon of biceps in the cubital fossa
C The anterior tibial artery is palpable at the ankle midway between the malleoli
D The facial artery can be palpated against the mandible at the anterior edge of the masseter muscle
E The dorsalis pedis artery runs medial to the tendon of extensor hallucis longus on the dorsum of the foot

13. **Regarding physiological differences between adults and infants**

A   Neonates have a higher body water content than adults
B   Neonates are more susceptible to temperature changes due to their larger relative surface area and immature control mechanisms
C   The only mature organ at birth is the liver
D   Neonates require an operating theatre temperature of less than 27°C
E   The heart rate of a neonate is nearly double that of a healthy adult

14. **Constituents of bile**

A   Include cholesterol
B   Have the same concentration throughout the biliary tree
C   Primary bile contains sodium at a concentration of 70–80 mmol/l
D   Bile pigments account for the largest portion of dry mass
E   There are few or no chloride ions in bile

15. **Carcinoma of the prostate**

A   Is caused by industrial dyes
B   Is mainly 'squamous cell' in type
C   Is graded according to Clark's score
D   Commonly metastasizes to bone
E   Has a stable incidence over the age of 55

16. **Liver abscesses**

A   May be caused by amoeba
B   The infecting organism in hydatid disease is a fungus
C   May rupture into the bronchial tree
D   Hydatid disease is mediated by fresh water snails
E   May be a complication of cholangiocarcinoma

17. **Regarding hallux valgus**

A   It is more frequently seen in females
B   The first metatarsal is usually normally aligned
C   Metatarsalgia is almost never present
D   A bunion is an exostosis formed over the most medial point of the deformity
E   It is associated with second toe abnormalities

18. The subclavian steal syndrome

A Presents as amaurosis fugax on walking
B Causes dizziness on exercising the arm with the affected subclavian artery
C The causative lesion is atherosclerosis of the 2nd part of the subclavian
D A supraclavicular bruit may be audible on auscultation
E The condition can be diagnosed by showing reversed flow in the vertebral artery on exercising the limb

19. Regarding hypertrophic pyloric stenosis

A It occurs more commonly in boys
B It presents with projectile bilious vomiting
C It typically presents in the third month of life
D The diagnosis can be made using USS
E The neonate may have metabolic acidosis

20. Abdominal stomas

A Result in weight loss
B Are not useful in ileoanal anastomoses
C Can be complicated by parastomal hernia
D Can be associated with increased incidence of gallstones
E When fashioned in the right iliac fossa usually indicate transverse loop colostomy

21. Testicular cancer

A Is associated with undescended testis -
B Is most likely to be a teratoma in a 19-year-old patient
C α-Fetoprotein is elevated in the majority of cases of seminoma
D Adjuvant therapy is usually needed for patients with disease confined to the testis
E Spreads to the inguinal lymph nodes

22. Complications of fractures include

A Reflex sympathetic dystrophy
B Pneumothorax
C Fat embolism
D Neurological deficit
E Osteoarthritis
F Compartment syndrome

23. **The short saphenous vein**

A   Drains the lateral venous plexus on the dorsum of the foot
B   Is closely related to the sural nerve
C   Starts in front of the lateral malleolus
D   Does not communicate with the long saphenous vein
E   Terminates in the popliteal fossa

24. **Hirschsprung's disease**

A   Is an aquired condition
B   May be associated with Down's syndrome
C   Is aganglionosis of the distal colon and rectum
D   Surgical treatment is by Ramstedt's procedure
E   Is not associated with colorectal cancer

25. **Child's criteria for assessment of portal hypertension include**

A   Age
B   Bleeding time
C   Serum albumin
D   Ascites
E   Alkaline phosphatase

26. **Humeral supracondylar fractures**

A   Commonly occur in adults
B   If malunited can result in cubitus varus
C   The displacement of the distal fragment is usually anterior and medial
D   Alignment should be sought even if the pulse is no longer palpable as this returns once the plaster cast is applied
E   Median nerve injury is a recognized complication

27. **A carotid body tumour**

A   Is also called chemodectoma
B   Is malignant in 90% of cases
C   Arises about 2.5 cm above the medial end of the clavicle

D Causes a splayed appearance of the internal and external carotid arteries on arteriography

E On clinical examination the lump can be moved from side to side but not up and down

F Is compressible

28. The adrenal glands

A The left gland is supplied by one suprarenal artery which is a branch of the aorta

B The right gland lies against the bare area of the liver

C The glands are covered by the renal fascia anteriorly only

D The left gland drains into the inferior vena cava via the left suprarenal vein

E The right gland drains directly into the portal vein

29. Inguinal hernia in infants

A Is associated with a patent processus vaginalis

B Occurs most commonly in boys

C May be treated in gallows traction if incarcerated

D Presents most commonly after the second year of life

30. Pancreatic cancer

A Has an increasing incidence

B Occurs most commonly in females

C Is commonly squamous cell carcinoma

D Occurs most commonly in the head and neck of the gland

E 60% of patients have localized disease at presentation which is 'curable' by resection

31. Ankle injuries

A Fractures of the ankle are classified according to Neer's classification

B A fracture of the lateral malleolus below the tibiofibular joint can be managed in a plaster cast

C Swelling of the ankle should not delay operative treatment if indicated

D A fibular fracture above the tibiofibular ligament with talar shift should be manipulated under anaesthetic and the reduction held using a plaster cast

E It is usually advisable to fix a bimalleolar fracture internally

32. Blood pressure

A   Is the systemic vascular resistance divided by cardiac output
B   Is directly proportional to stroke volume
C   The mean arterial pressure is closer in value to the diastolic than the systolic pressure
D   Is regulated by baroreceptors

33. Tracheostomy

A   Is indicated in a trauma patient with severe facial injuries
B   May be complicated by tracheal stenosis
C   Can help increase ventilatory dead space
D   Affords easy access to the bronchotracheal tree for lavage
E   A fistula between the trachea and the right atrium is a recognized complication

34. Inguinal hernias

A   Are more common on the right than the left side by a ratio of 5:2
B   Are indirect in females
C   Are twice as common as femoral hernias in females
D   Have the same incidence in male and female infants
E   Are associated with aortic aneurysms

35. Renal calculi

A   The incidence rises with age
B   Are associated with secondary hyperparathyroidism
C   *Proteus* infection results in triple phosphate stones
D   The pelvic brim is a common site for stone hold up
E   Have a similar incidence in males and females

36. The hip joint

A   Can be approached posteriorly by dividing the piriformis, obturator internus and gemelli
B   The femoral nerve supplies the muscles that cause flexion
C   Adduction is performed by muscles innervated by S1
D   The articular surface of the acetabulum is doughnut shaped
E   The iliofemoral ligament prevents hyperextension

37. Buerger's disease

A   Has a predilection for medium-sized arteries
B   Affects smokers and non-smokers with the same frequency
C   Frequently presents with digital infections and gangrene
D   Sympathectomy is rarely beneficial in treating this condition
E   Bypass surgery is the main treatment

38. Pharyngeal pouch

A   Is a diverticulum between the muscles of the middle pharyngeal constrictor
B   May present with recurrent pneumonia
C   May be palpable on the left side of the neck below the thyroid cartilage
D   Is frequently seen in middle-aged males
E   The diverticulum may contain a carcinoma

39. The following layers are incised in a vertical paramedian laparotomy incision

A   Scarpa's fascia
B   Transversus fascia
C   Anterior rectus sheath
D   Linea alba
E   Linea semilunaris
F   Visceral peritoneum

40. Bladder diverticulum

A   May be congenital
B   Is associated with urinary tract infection
C   May predispose to adenocarcinoma of the bladder
D   Is best investigated using IVU
E   Is associated with stone formation

41. Osteomyelitis

A   Is most commonly caused by *Staphylococcus aureus*
B   Antibiotic therapy should be continued for 3 weeks
C   May be caused by *Salmonella* in children with sickle cell disease
D   When occurs postoperatively is almost always caused by *Bacteroides fragilis*
E   Is uncommon in children

42. **The following are recognized causes of aneurysm formation**

A Gonococcal infection
B Atherosclerosis
C Syphilis
D Collagen disorders
E Trauma

43. **The pharynx**

A Is composed of four constrictor muscles
B Is continuous with the oesophagus at its inferior end
C The thoracic duct passes in the retropharyngeal space
D Derives its motor supply from the accessory nerve via the vagus nerve
E Is surrounded by a ring of lymphoid tissue at the entrance to the aerodigestive tract

44. **Carcinoma of the anus**

A Metastasizes to the external iliac lymph nodes
B Is best treated with abdominoperineal resection
C May be predisposed to by human papilloma virus infection
D Can be treated with radiotherapy
E Is mostly of squamous cell origin

45. **Wilms' tumour**

A Has a peak incidence at the age of 2–3 years
B Is malignant in 50% of cases
C Is bilateral in 50% of cases
D May be familial
E Is also known as nephroblastoma

46. **The shoulder joint**

A Is an atypical synovial joint
B The synovial membrane invests the short head of the biceps in the intertubercular groove
C The joint is weakest inferiorly
D The median nerve is closely related to the joint inferiorly and should be examined after anterior dislocation
E The axillary nerve supplies the deltoid muscle which abducts the shoulder

47. The carotid artery

A The internal carotid artery has two important branches in the neck
B The first branch of the external carotid artery is the superior thyroid artery
C Is enclosed by the carotid sheath together with the internal jugular vein and the phrenic nerve
D Bifurcates at the level of the cricoid cartilage
E Is deep to the ansa cervicalis

48. The recurrent laryngeal nerve

A Is the laryngeal branch of the glossolaryngeal nerve
B 'Recurs' around the subclavian artery on the right
C Supplies sensation of the whole of the larynx
D The left recurrent laryngeal nerve arises in the thorax and 'recurs' around the arch of the aorta
E Supplies the majority of the intrinsic muscles of the larynx

49. The following are known risk factors for developing oesophageal cancer

A Gastro-oesophageal reflux
B Achalasia
C Barrett's oesophagus
D Lye stricture
E Nitrosamines

50. Torsion of the testis

A Has a peak incidence around the age of 15
B Is associated with undescended testis
C Is associated with a long testicular mesentery
D Can be diagnosed using duplex scanning
E The affected testis lies higher than the normal one

EMQs

Theme: Foot operations

Options:
a Proximal interphalangeal joint fusion
b Keller's operation
c Forefoot arthroplasty

d First metatarsal osteotomy
e Cheilectomy
f Arthrodesis
g Tendon transfer

For each of the case scenarios below, choose the single most likely option from the list above. Each option may be used once, more than once or not at all.

61. A 55-year-old female journalist presents with bilateral symptomatic hallux valgus.
62. A 60-year-old male complains of a painful right second toe. On examination he has a fixed flexed proximal toe joint and fixed extended distal joint.
63. A 70-year-old patient presents with severely symptomatic hallux valgus.
64. A 25-year-old dancer presents with a painful rigid first metatarsophalangeal joint.

Theme: Leg ulcers

Options:
a Ischaemic ulcers
b Venous ulcers
c Pyoderma gangrenosum
d Marjolin's ulcer
e Rheumatoid ulcer
f Neuropathic ulcers
g Basal cell carcinoma
h Sickle cell disease ulcer

For each of the case scenarios below, choose the single most likely option from the list above. Each option may be used once, more than once or not at all.

65. A 65-year-old woman presents with a swollen right leg and a 5-cm diameter ulcer above the medial malleolus. Her leg has been intermittently swollen for the last 10 years. The sensation and pulses are normal.
66. A woman presents with a progressively worsening leg ulcer. She has had it for 7 years and was looked after by her GP and district nurse. On examination she has a foul-smelling ulcer with heaped-up edges.
67. A patient presents with a 2-week history of leg ulcer. On examination the ulcer appears to have a black sloughy edge but the neurovascular status of the legs is normal.
68. An elderly man presents with a deep ulcer over the heel. Examination reveals normal pulses.

Theme: Abnormalities of calcium metabolism

Options:

a   Vitamin D intoxication
b   Primary hyperparathyroidism
c   Secondary hyperparathyroidism
d   Tertiary hyperparathyroidism
e   Multiple meyloma
f   Bone metastases
g   Paget's disease
h   Sarcoid

For each of the case scenarios below, choose the single most likely option from the list above. Each option may be used once, more than once or not at all.

69. A 33-year-old insulin-dependent diabetic is admitted with abdominal pain and vomiting. He has recently received a renal transplant having been dependent on dialysis for the last 5 years. His amylase is 800 iu/l, calcium 3.1 mmol/l, phosphate 1.6 mmol/l (reference range 0.8–1.4 mmol/l) and PTH 280 ng/l (reference range 10–65 ng/l).
70. A 65-year-old female is admitted with back pain. Her serum calcium is 3.3 mmol/l, alkaline phosphatase 360 iu/l, and her urine contains Bence-Jones proteins.
71. A 43-year-old female is admitted with recurrent ureteric colic. Her serum calcium is 3.4 mmol/l, phosphate 0.7 mmol/l and PTH 170 ng/l.

Theme: Painful inguinoscrotal swellings in childhood

Options:

a   Strangulated inguinal hernia
b   Rectus sheath haematoma
c   Epididymitis
d   Hydrocele
e   Torsion of the testis
f   Incarcerated femoral hernia
g   Torsion of hydatid of Morgagni
h   Maldescent of the testis (in the inguinal canal)

For each of the case scenarios below, choose the single most likely option from the list above. Each option may be used once, more than once or not at all.

72. A 5-year-old boy complains of severe pain in the groin following trauma to the area while playing. Examination reveals a tender lump above and lateral to the pubic tubercle.
73. A 13-year-old boy presents with scrotal pain. On examination there is no swelling or erythema of the scrotum. The left testis is tender with a small palpable mass at the upper pole.

74. A 12-year-old boy presents with acute right scrotal pain, and nausea and vomiting. This has been present for 3 hours. He is difficult to examine as he has a tense and extremely tender scrotum.

Theme: Oesophageal conditions

Options:
a   Mallory–Weiss syndrome
b   Achalasia
c   Scleroderma
d   Oesophageal rupture
e   Carcinoma of the oesophagus
f   Peptic stricture
g   Candidiasis
h   Zenker's diverticulum

For each of the case scenarios below, choose the single most likely option from the list above. Each option may be used once, more than once or not at all.

75. A 47-year-old man is brought to A&E from a party where he had excessive amounts of food and wine. He is complaining of severe chest pain which started following an episode of vomiting. Clinically he is shocked with epigastric rigidity.
76. A 52-year-old diabetic patient presents with excessive pain and difficulty swallowing. Her diabetes is reasonably controlled on insulin but she has retinopathy and received a cadaveric renal transplant 2 years ago.
77. A 45-year-old woman is investigated for dysphagia and recurrent pneumonia using oesophageal manometry. This shows a high resting pressure in the lower oesophageal sphincter which fails to relax, and absence of peristalsis in the body of the oesophagus.
78. A 63-year-old woman with dysphagia is investigated using manometry. This shows normal peristalsis in the upper third but little activity in the lower two thirds of the oesophagus.

Theme: Venous conditions

Options:
a   Aspirin
b   Thromboembolic prophylaxis using stockings, heparin, etc.
c   Life-long warfarin
d   Embolectomy
e   Thrombolysis
f   Caval filter
g   Standard heparin in three daily doses for 6 weeks

For each of the case scenarios below, choose the single most likely option from the list above. Each option may be used once, more than once or not at all.

79. A 72-year-old woman was admitted with a cerebrovascular accident. Initially she was unable to swallow but her symptoms are now resolving. A duplex scan of her swollen leg showed an iliofemoral deep vein thrombosis.

80. A 42-year-old male with a family history of deep vein thrombosis presents with a second episode of proximal leg vein thrombosis.

81. A 65-year-old woman is admitted for a right hemicolectomy. She had a pulmonary embolus 6 years ago following which she was on warfarin for 6 months.

Theme: Jaundice

Options:

a   Head of pancreas carcinoma
b   Gallstones in the common bile duct
c   Gilbert syndrome
d   Sclerosing cholangitis
e   Viral hepatitis
f   Haemolytic anaemia
g   Primary biliary cirrhosis
h   Alcoholic liver disease

For each of the case scenarios below, choose the single most likely option from the list above. Each option may be used once, more than once or not at all.

82. A 25-year-old Caucasian male presents with recurrent attacks of mild jaundice. These are not associated with any other symptoms. His liver function tests are normal except for bilirubin of 35 μmol/l.

83. A 55-year-old homeless man with a history of alcohol abuse presents with progressive jaundice and weight loss. He also complains of passing dark urine and light-coloured stools, and severe epigastric pain radiating to the back.

84. A 30-year-old woman presents with a 1-week history of right upper quadrant pain, fever and jaundice. She has tender hepatomegaly and her liver function tests show a bilirubin of 75 μmol/l, ALP of 300 iu/l and AST of 2500 iu/l.

Theme: Urinary incontinence

Options:

a   Chronic incontinence
b   Overflow incontinence
c   Stress incontinence
d   Active incontinence
e   Urge incontinence
f   Passive incontinence
g   Obstructive incontinence

For each of the case scenarios below, choose the single most likely option from the list above. Each option may be used once, more than once or not at all.

85. A 73-year-old man attends routine follow-up after TURP. He complains of passing water every time he coughs or strains.
86. A 79-year-old man presents with bed wetting. He used to get up four times a night to pass urine. He suddenly started to wet his bed at night 2 weeks ago.
87. An Ethiopian immigrant mother of four attends clinic complaining of incontinence. On further questioning, through an interpreter, she mentions the passage of urine per vagina.

Theme: Carcinoma of the prostate

Options:
a   External beam radiotherapy
b   Combination chemotherapy
c   Expectant policy
d   Prostatectomy
e   Gonadotrophin-releasing hormone analogue
f   Laser
g   Transurethral resection of the prostate

For each of the case scenarios below, choose the single most likely option from the list above. Each option may be used once, more than once or not at all.

88. A 54-year-old patient presents with carcinoma of the prostate. The disease is thought to be confined to the prostate.
89. Mr Nelson is 74 years of age. He was attending routine follow-up clinic for prostatic carcinoma when he complained of back pain. A bone scan arranged at the last visit shows skeletal metastases.
90. A 72-year-old man was found to have well-differentiated malignant cells after examining prostatic chips from a recent TURP. A bone scan is negative.

Theme: Management of urinary tract calculi

Options:
a   Cystostomy
b   Ureteric stenting
c   Extracorporeal shockwave lithotripsy (ESWL)
d   Nephrostomy
e   Analgesia
f   Ureteroscopy and ESWL (push-bang)
g   Percutaneous nephrolithotomy

For each of the case scenarios below, choose the single most likely option from the list above. Each option may be used once, more than once or not at all.

91. A 32-year-old man was admitted with ureteric colic 48 hours previously. An IVU reveals an 8 mm stone in the upper third of the ureter and hydronephrosis.
92. A 35-year-old man is known to have a 3 cm stone in the renal pelvis. Two previous attempts at ESWL failed to break up this calculus. He is still symptomatic.
93. A 26-year-old woman presents with a severe left-sided abdominal pain and vomiting. A plain radiograph and an IVU show a 4 mm calculus at the pelvic rim.

Theme: Hip conditions

Options:
a Septic arthritis
b Rheumatoid arthritis
c Perthe's
d Slipped upper femoral epiphysis
e Congenital dislocation
f Irritable hip
g Fractured neck of femur

For each of the case scenarios below, choose the single most likely option from the list above. Each option may be used once, more than once or not at all.

94. An 18-month-old infant is systemically unwell for 24 hours. She stopped walking and is reluctant to move her right leg. She also has a fever.
95. A 5-year-old boy presents with a 9-day history of painful left hip. He also developed a limp. On examination there is reduction in all hip movements. X-ray films of the hip show increased density of the epiphysis.
96. Jonathan is a 14-year-old prepubertal boy presenting with a 3-month history of painful right hip and limping. On examination he appears obese and has a slightly shorter and externally rotated right leg.

Theme: Peripheral nerve injuries in the lower limb

Options:
a S1
b L4
c L5
d Common peroneal nerve
e Superficial peroneal nerve
f Sciatic nerve
g Femoral nerve

For each of the case scenarios below, choose the single most likely option from the list above. Each option may be used once, more than once or not at all.

97. A patient presents with loss of sensation over the front and lateral side of his leg and foot. There is no foot drop but he is unable to evert his foot.
98. A patient presents with loss of sensation over the front of the foot and leg. He is unable to extend the big toe.
99. A patient presents with loss of sensation over the sole of the foot, reduced power on plantar flexion and reduced ankle reflex.
100. A patient presents with loss of sensation over the front and lateral side of the leg and the dorsum of the foot. She also has weakness on dorsiflexion and eversion of the foot.

Theme: Visual field deficit

Options:
a   Retinal detachment
b   Transection of the optic nerve
c   Pituitary tumour
d   Transection of the right optic tract
e   A lesion affecting the optic radiation
f   Right occipital cortex infarcts
g   Transection of the left optic tract

For each of the case scenarios below, choose the single most likely option from the list above. Each option may be used once, more than once or not at all.

101. A patient with bitemporal hemianopia.
102. A patient with left homonymous hemianopia with macular sparing.

Theme: The acute abdomen

Options:
a   Perforated peptic ulcer
b   Acute cholecystitis
c   Acute appendicitis
d   Intestinal obstruction
e   Strangulated hernia
f   Acute pancreatitis
g   Intestinal ischaemia

For each of the case scenarios below, choose the single most likely option from the list above. Each option may be used once, more than once or not at all.

103. A 28-year-old female presents with pain in the epigastrium. On examination she is febrile and has localized tenderness in the right hypochondrium.

104. A 73-year-old man is brought to A&E. He has been unwell for 8 hours. His main complaint is abdominal pain which has changed from intermittent to constant and vomiting brown blood-stained liquid vomitus. Previously he was healthy except for 'stomach ulcer' surgery 30 years ago. He has a pulse of 110 bpm and systolic pressure of 90 mmHg. A blood gas analysis shows him to have metabolic acidosis. There are distended small bowel loops on the X-ray but no free gas under the diaphragm.

105. A 32-year-old male presents with a 6-hour history of epigastric abdominal pain. He is known to have been HIV positive for the last 7 years and was started on triple anti-HIV therapy 3 weeks ago. He has signs of peritonism in the epigastrium but no free gas on the erect chest X-ray.

ANSWERS TO PRACTICE PAPER THREE

The letters of the correct answers are given

MCQs

1. Regarding muscles that act on the fingers
A, C, D, E
The lateral two lumbricals are supplied by the median nerve. The medial two are supplied by the ulnar nerve.

2. The femoral triangle
All true

3. Clinical diagnosis of varicose veins
B, E
A venous thrill on coughing indicates saphenofemoral incompetence. Ulceration occurs in the gaiter area when associated with varicose veins. The diagnosis of perforator incompetence cannot be made from the distribution of varicosities.

4. Complications of pancreatitis
B, C
ARDS occurs in the presence of pulmonary artery wedge pressure (i.e. left atrial pressure) of less than 18 mmHg. Patients with pancreatitis have large fluid deficits; therefore, active replacement to maintain adequate urine output is mandatory.

5. Renal trauma
All true
Renal trauma can result in a retroperitoneal haematoma. This is a classic cause of paralytic ileus.

6. The cubital fossa
A, C, E
The cubital fossa is bounded by pronator teres medially and brachioradialis laterally. Its contents from medial to lateral are the median nerve, the brachial artery and the tendon of the biceps. The radial nerve runs laterally under the edge of brachioradialis.

7. The thoracic inlet
D, E, F
The scalene muscles are covered by prevertebral fascia. The subclavian artery and the three trunks of the brachial plexus emerge between the scalenus anterior and medius muscles carrying an extension of fascia with them called the axillary sheath. This does

not cover the vein as it emerges anterior to scalenus anterior and therefore anterior to the prevertebral fascia. T1 root joins C8 to form the inferior trunk of the brachial plexus and passes over the 1st rib to enter the axilla.

8.   Phaeochromocytoma
D, E
Phaeochromocytoma is bilateral in 10%, malignant in 10% and familial in 10%. The tumour can be diagnosed by measuring plasma catecholamine and urinary VMA levels. MRI, CT and nuclear isotope scanning are used to localize it.

9.   Gastric acid secretion is stimulated by
A, C, E
Gastric secretion is stimulated by both neuronal and hormonal mechanisms. The vagus stimulates oxyntic glands using acetylcholine as a neurotransmitter. Food entering the stomach stimulates G cells which produce gastrin. This reaches the oxyntic and peptic cells via the blood stream. The secretory glands also have histamine receptors.

10.   Urodynamic studies
A, B

Compliance = Δ Pressure/Δ Volume

When performing a urodynamic study pressure probes are inserted into the bladder and the rectum.

Detrusor pressure = Intravesical pressure − Rectal pressure

Uroflowmetry also measures the total urinary volume.

11.   Paget's disease of the bone
B, D, E
Paget's disease is common in Caucasians. The biochemical abnormality is elevated alkaline phosphatase.

12.   Surface anatomy of some palpable pulses
C, D
The femoral artery enters the lower limb at the midinguinal point and can be palpated here. The brachial artery is medial to the tendon of biceps in the cubital fossa and dorsalis pedis is lateral to the tendon of extensor hallucis longus on the dorsum of the foot.

13.   Regarding physiological differences between adults and infants
A, B, E
The neonate's physiological function and control are immature at birth. The liver's synthetic, metabolic and storage functions are underdeveloped at birth. The minimum required theatre temperature is above 30°C.

14. Constituents of bile
A only

Bile contains bile salts, lecithins and bile pigments. Primary bile contains the aforementioned in a fluid similar to plasma in its electrolyte content. Bile salts account for about 50% of dry mass.

15. Carcinoma of the prostate
D only

Prostatic carcinoma is a common disease in older men and its incidence rises with age to nearly 80% in men over the age of 80. Most tumours are adenocarcinomas and are graded using Gleason's system. This correlates well with prognosis.

16. Liver abscesses
A, C, E

Hydatid disease is most commonly seen in sheep rearing areas. It is caused by the parasite *Echinococcus granulosus* for which the dog is the most common host.

17. Regarding hallux valgus
A, E

Hallux valgus is caused by medial deviation of the first metatarsal (metatarsus primus varus) and valgus deviation of the big toe. It often causes pain and the bunion, which is a bursa, may become inflamed. The second toe is often overriding and may become 'hammer' or 'mallet'.

18. The subclavian steal syndrome
A, D, E

This condition results from occlusion of the 1st part of the subclavian artery proximal to the origin of the vertebral artery. Increased demand for blood supply to the arm leads to a steal phenomenon from the circle of Willis down the vertebral artery, which is a branch of the 1st part of the subclavian, and into the subclavian artery distal to the stenosis.

19. Regarding hypertrophic pyloric stenosis
A, D

This condition has an incidence of about 4 in 1000 live births. It is more common in Caucasians and about 15% of cases have a family history. The condition usually presents in the first month of life and the vomitus is typically not bile stained. There may be metabolic alkalosis and hypokalaemia.

20. Abdominal stomas
C, D

A loop ileostomy fashioned at the time of low anterior resection of the rectum reduces the complications from anastomotic leaks. A stoma in the right iliac fossa usually indicates a loop or end ileostomy.

21. Testicular cancer
A, B, D

α-Fetoprotein and/or βhCG are elevated in a large proportion of patients with teratoma whereas βhCG is raised in a minority of patients with seminoma.

Lymphatic spread is to the para-aortic nodes; therefore, the inguinal nodes are only involved if the tumour invades the scrotal skin.

22. Complications of fractures include
All true

23. The short saphenous vein
A, B, E

The short saphenous vein commences posterior to the lateral malleolus and courses on the back of the calf towards the popliteal fossa. Before terminating there it usually communicates with the long saphenous vein through a variable number of branches.

24. Hirschsprung's disease
B, C, E

This is a congenital condition which affects boys more than girls. Its surgical management encompasses Duhamel's, Soave's and Swenson's procedures. Ramstedt's procedure is employed in the treatment of hypertrophic pyloric stenosis.

25. Child's criteria for assessment of portal hypertension include
C, D

The other criteria are serum bilirubin, prothrombin time and encephalopathy.

26. Humeral supracondylar fractures
B, E

This fracture is more common in children. The fracture is usually treated by reduction under anaesthesia and collar and cuff; it may also require pin fixation. Recognition and treatment of neurovascular injury is paramount.

27. A carotid body tumour
A, D, E, F

Carotid body tumours are usually unilateral and are malignant in about 5% of cases although this is difficult to quantify. The tumour arises at the level of the bifurcation of the carotid, i.e. the upper border of the thyroid cartilage.

28. The adrenal glands
B only

The glands are enclosed by the renal fascia where they have a separate compartment. The glands are supplied by three arteries each: the superior suprarenal is a branch of the inferior phrenic artery, the middle suprarenal is a direct branch of the aorta and the inferior suprarenal is a branch of the renal artery. The right adrenal drains blood directly into the vena cava but the left drains into the ipsilateral renal vein, as does the left testis.

29. Inguinal hernia in infants
A, B, C
This condition presents most commonly in the first 2 years of life.

30. Pancreatic cancer
A, D
Pancreatic carcinoma has a M:F ratio of 1. The most common histological type is adenocarcinoma. Only about 20% of cases present at a resectable stage.

31. Ankle injuries
B, E
Ankle fractures can be classified according to Weber's classification: fibular fractures at the level of the syndesmosis are type B, below it are type A and above it are type C. Unstable injuries involving the syndesmosis or those causing derangement of the mortise are usually treated operatively. In the presence of excessive swelling, surgery is deferred for a few days until this subsides.

32. Blood pressure
B, C, D

$$BP = CO \times SVR$$

$$CO = SV \times HR$$

$$BP_{mean} = BP_{diastolic} + 1/3 \, (BP_{systolic} - BP_{diastolic})$$

33. Tracheostomy
A, B, D
Tracheostomy reduces the anatomical dead space.
The trachea is not anatomically related to the right atrium but a fistula with the brachiocephalic artery is a recognized complication of tracheostomy.

34. Inguinal hernias
B, E
The ratio of R:L is 5:4. Inguinal and femoral hernias have a similar incidence in females. However, direct inguinal hernias are rare in females. Male infants are about eight to nine times more likely to have a hernia than a female infant. There is a higher incidence in premature babies, low-birth-weight babies and twins.

35. Renal calculi
C, D
Renal calculi are four times more common in males than females. They mostly occur in early adult life with a peak in the late twenties and again in the mid-fifties. Common sites for hold up are the pelviureteric junction, the pelvic brim and the vesicoureteric junction.

36. The hip joint
A, B, E
The adductor muscles are supplied by the obturator nerve which has the same root value as the femoral nerve, i.e. L2, 3, 4. The articular surface is horseshoe shaped.

37. Buerger's disease
A, C
This condition affects young males who are heavy smokers and usually affects medium-sized arteries. Bypass surgery is often difficult due to the nature of the distal vessels; therefore, treatment is usually focused on giving up smoking, sympathectomy and amputation.

38. Pharyngeal pouch
B, C, E
Incoordination of pharyngeal muscle activity leads to diverticulum formation in Killian's dehiscence which is a space between the muscles of the inferior constrictor. This condition is most commonly seen in the elderly and usually presents with dysphagia.

39. The following layers are incised in a vertical paramedian laparotomy incision
A, B, C

40. Bladder diverticulum
A, B, E
Stones developing in the diverticulum and chronic inflammation predispose to squamous cell carcinoma. The best method for demonstrating a diverticulum is by performing a micturating cystogram.

41. Osteomyelitis
A, C
This condition is more common in childhood. Postoperatively it is usually caused by *Proteus, Pseudomonas* and *Staphylococcus epidermidis* and *aureus*. Treatment with antibiotics should be given for a minimum of 6 weeks.

42. The following are recognized causes of aneurysm formation
B, C, D, E
Syphilis is a very rare cause now. Another cause is congenital weakness of the wall of the artery.

43. The pharynx
B, D, E
The pharynx is made up of the superior, middle and inferior constrictors. Behind it is the retropharyngeal space, which is loose connective tissue where infection can spread rapidly.

44. Carcinoma of the anus

C, D, E

Squamous cell carcinoma of the anus usually metastasizes to the inguinal lymph nodes. Abdominoperineal resection is no longer the primary treatment modality for this condition. Radiotherapy and chemoradiation have, by and large, replaced surgery.

45. Wilms' tumour

C, E

This is the commonest renal malignancy in childhood and accounts for 10% of all childhood malignancies. Only 5% of cases are bilateral.

46. The shoulder joint

C, E

The shoulder joint is a typical synovial joint of the ball-and-socket type. The synovium invests the long head of the biceps. The axillary nerve lies close to the inferior aspect of the joint and can be injured in anterior dislocation.

47. The carotid artery

B, E

The common carotid artery bifurcates at the level of the upper border of the thyroid cartilage. The internal carotid has no branches in the neck. The carotid sheath contains the common carotid artery, the internal jugular vein and the vagus nerve.

48. The recurrent laryngeal nerve

B, D, E

The recurrent laryngeal nerve is a branch of the vagus nerve. The right arises in the neck and hooks around the right subclavian artery; the left arises in the thorax. They both head towards the larynx in the tracheo-oesophageal groove. They supply all the intrinsic muscles of the larynx except the cricothyroid muscle. The sensory supply is to the mucous membrane below the vocal cords.

49. The following are known risk factors for developing oesophageal cancer

B, C, D, E

Gastro-oesophageal reflux is not a risk factor unless it develops into a stricture or Barrett's oesophagus.

50. Torsion of the testis

All true

EMQs

Theme: Foot operations

61-d This is the operative treatment of choice for the younger more mobile patient.

62-a This is claw toe. It is treated by excising the corn that forms over the PIP joint and fusing the joint using a K-wire.

63-b Hallux valgus in the elderly patient should be treated conservatively if possible. A Keller's operation may be considered in cases which do not respond to conservative treatment.

64-e Hallux rigidus is the likely cause of this patient's complaint. Cheilectomy involves the removal of a dorsal segment of the metatarsal head and osteophytes.

Theme: Leg ulcers

65-b This is compatible with venous ulceration. The swollen leg may be secondary to missed deep vein thrombosis.

66-d This is a squamous cell carcinoma which developed in a chronic venous ulcer.

67-c The short history, black slough and otherwise normal examination point to this condition.

68-f Deep ulcers over pressure areas in the absence of clinical signs of ischaemia make this diagnosis most likely.

Theme: Abnormalities of calcium metabolism

69-d Unlike primary hyperparathyroidism the fasting phosphate may be elevated. Autonomous PTH secretion, thought to result in response to chronic hypocalcaemia, coupled with the new kidney's ability to metabolize vitamin D results in this condition.

70-e Bone malignancies are a common cause of hypercalcaemia.

71-b This condition occurs as a result of parathyroid hyperplasia or an adenoma. Rarely, this condition can be caused by a parathyroid carcinoma.

Theme: Painful inguinoscrotal swellings in childhood

72-h This is the commonest site for a maldescended testis.

73-g

74-e Remember that torsion is much more common in the age group 5 to about 15.

Theme: Oesophageal conditions

75-d This condition can be confused with a dissecting aneurysm or myocardial infarction. The cardiovascular collapse results from chemical mediastinitis. There may be clinical and radiological evidence of gas in the mediastinum and subcutaneous tissue.

76-g Fungal and viral infections usually occur in immune deficiency and patients on immunosuppressive drugs.

77-b Achalasia is an uncommon condition affecting 1 in 100 000. It is physiologically characterized by the manometric findings above.

78-c These are typical manometric findings in scleroderma.

Theme: Venous conditions
79-f Anti-coagulation in any form carries a risk of a haemorrhagic stroke. A caval filter will reduce the risk of pulmonary embolus and avoid the risks of anti-coagulation.

80-c Recurrent thromboembolism is an indication for life-long anti-coagulation.

81-b Thromboembolic prophylaxis is the norm in surgical practice nowadays. She ought to have been investigated for thrombophilia at some stage following her pulmonary embolus.

Theme: Jaundice
82-c

83-a

84-e The highly elevated transaminase, fever and hepatomegaly favour acute viral hepatitis.

Theme: Urinary incontinence
85-c Sphincter weakness in men is uncommon but can follow prostatectomy

86-b This patient with chronic retention has developed overflow incontinence.

87-f A vesicovaginal fistula presents with passive incontinence.

Theme: Carcinoma of the prostate
88-d Confined disease in a young patient is best treated by surgery.

89-e Metastatic disease is treated by hormonal manipulation. Gonadotrophin-releasing hormone is one of many modalities.

90-c This type of patient is usually treated expectantly. If the tumour grade is less differentiated then radiotherapy may be given.

Theme: Management of urinary tract calculi
91-f The calculus is first pushed back into the renal pelvis. This is followed by lithotripsy.

92-g

93-e It is likely that this stone will pass spontaneously as it is less than 5 mm in diameter.

Theme: Hip conditions
94-a

95-c This condition affects the age group 4–8 years. The immediate treatment should concentrate on rest, skin traction and analgesia while the hip is painful.

96-d This is a fairly typical presentation of this condition which affects children around puberty. There may also be a history of trauma to the hip. Treatment aims at preventing further slip.

Theme: Peripheral nerve injuries in the lower limb

97-e This nerve supplies the peroneal muscles, hence the loss of eversion. It should be differentiated from common peroneal nerve injury which involves loss of function of both superficial and deep peroneal nerves. The deep peroneal nerve supplies the anterior compartment of the leg. Its injury causes inability to dorsiflex the foot.

98-c This is the sensory and motor deficit which is characteristic of L5 root injury.

99-a This is characteristic of deficit of this nerve root.

100-d

Theme: Visual field deficit

101-c Lesions affecting the visual fields in both eyes are usually in the optic chiasma, the optic tracts or more proximally. Pressure on the nerve fibres, which lie in the centre of the chiasma as they cross over to the contralateral optic tract, from the nasal side of the retina causes bilateral temporal field deficit.

102-f Loss of one half of the visual field is caused by any postchiasmal lesion, i.e. tract, radiation or cortex. Macular sparing is characteristic of cortical blindness. The lesion is always on the opposite side of the visual deficit.

Theme: The acute abdomen

103-b

104-g The patient is gravely unwell. This diagnosis should be entertained in any patient who is very unwell in the face of paucity of abdominal signs. The adhesive obstruction has progressed into ischaemic gangrene.

105-f The newer anti-HIV drugs DDI and DDC are potent causes of acute pancreatitis. Serum amylase estimation will help make the diagnosis.